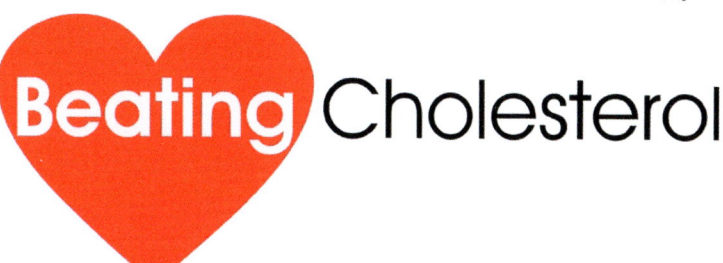

Beating Cholesterol

No Drugs,
No Secret Formula,
Simply Beat it the Natural Way . . .

Stephen Guy-Clarke

Published by Unity Health Centre
Beating Cholesterol

Copyright ©2016
All rights reserved.
No part of this book may be reproduced, stored in a retrieval system, or transmitted by any means, electronic, mechanical, photocopying, recording, or otherwise, without written permission from the copyright holder.

Typesetting & Cover Design by Ramesh Kumar Pitchai
ISBN 13: 978-1-52339-079-3
ISBN 10: 1-52339-079-4

First Edition 2006

Table of Contents

Acknowledgements 5

Introduction 6

Chapter 1 Cholesterol - what does it do and what makes it too high? Plus Triglycerides explained. 7

Chapter 2 What are the implications for health? 18

Chapter 3 What is the conventional approach to treatment? 21

Chapter 4 What are the alternatives to conventional Medicine? What works and what should we avoid? 29

Chapter 5 How you can beat High Cholesterol. 86

Action Plan 95

Further Reading 97

Recommended Listening 98

About the Author 99

References 100

Dedication

I dedicate this book to my late uncle, Bert Stonard. I feel his presence often with his incredible intellect and his gift for languages, a witty, compassionate, utterly positive man. Deeply spiritual, he meditated every day and his watchword was always 'To be in Tune with the Infinite'.

Today Friday 30th of July 2010 my dearest friend and business partner Justin Carter, whilst taking a cycle ride with his children Toby 11 and Freya 9 collapsed and died of a massive heart attack at the age of 56.

He leaves them and his loving wife Nancy.

'The Heavens shine brighter with Justin's light which touches us all'.

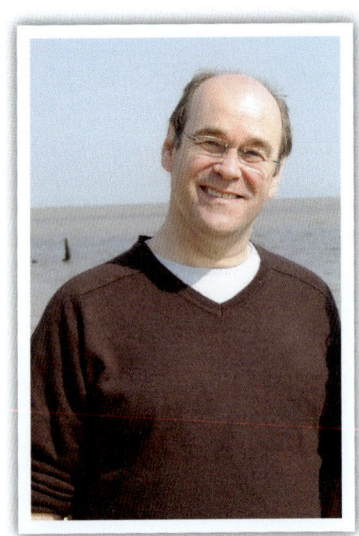

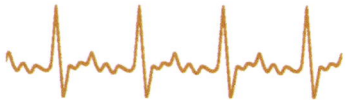

Acknowledgements

I owe my thanks to some very gifted people who have helped develop my passion for natural medicine. Firstly I thank my wife Christine for her insights and skills as a consummate natural health practitioner. Then I thank Dr Stephen Gascoigne for introducing me to Acupuncture, Dr John Stirling and Dr Gywnne Davies for their knowledge in naturopathic medicine, and Dr Gwynne Lewis for being a wonderful work colleague. Finally I thank all of my patients who have taught me about life.

Introduction

It is said that 'knowledge is power': when it is applied to one's health it can be truly 'empowering'.

How often do we talk about people being a 'victim of a heart attack'? The implication is that we are somehow 'ambushed' by this life threatening condition. It is my contention that the vast majority of cases of coronary artery disease are preventable if we take responsibility for our health and reduce the risk factors. This is the inspiration for this book, which is to enable you to make informed choices. Chapters 1 to 3 are self-explanatory, whereas chapter 4 can be read like a book or used as a reference guide to what works naturally and what to avoid. Chapter 5 has concise recommendations with a special section on an exciting Ayurvedic herb.

Wishing you vibrant health,

Stephen Guy Clarke

Chapter 1

Cholesterol – what does it do and what makes it too high?

Pick up any newspaper or magazine today and you will probably find mention of cholesterol. Our television screens and supermarket shelves are crying out with new products to combat the dangers of high cholesterol. Supermarkets like Tesco have gone one step further and decided to jump on the bandwagon and produce their own brand of cholesterol lowering products. The UK's biggest supermarket introduced its own plant sterol containing dairy range in January 2006. 'We've had so much interest in cholesterol lowering foods that we decided to launch our own range,' said Tesco. Multinationals such as Unilever, Danone and Coca-Cola are all promoting products with added plant sterols. Everyone seems to be concerned with lowering his or her cholesterol level and most people would like to know how they can do this safely without side effects.

Let's start by understanding how cholesterol is produced and used by the body.

Cholesterol is technically classified as a steroid, but is also classified as a lipid because it is soluble in fats. This crystalline substance is naturally found in the brain, nerves, liver, blood, and bile of humans. Despite all of the negative connotations, cholesterol is necessary for the proper functioning of the body. In fact your body can synthesise up to 1,500 milligrams of cholesterol a day (almost the amount in 10 eggs) using it for a number of crucial functions.

> (1) It serves as the precursor for bile acids that are formed in the liver and secreted in the bile to facilitate intestinal fat digestion.

(2) In the gonad and adrenal cortex, cholesterol is used to synthesise all steroid hormones.
(3) In the skin, it is used to form vitamin D3, a reaction requiring ultraviolet sun radiation.
(4) Cholesterol is found in abundance in the nerve tissue, where it is a component of the myelin sheath that electrically insulates the axons (the part of the nerve cell specialising in conducting impulses over large distances to other nerve, muscle, or gland cells).
(5) Cholesterol helps minimise evaporation of body water as well as making the skin waterproof.
(6) Last but not least, cholesterol is a stabilising component of the actual membranes of cells and their organelles (all cells contain 'miniorgans' called organelles, each specialised to perform a particular function, which is why liver cells differ from brain cells, which themselves differ from blood cells).

Hopefully you are now convinced that cholesterol is an essential substance in our body.

So where does cholesterol come from?

The answer lies in two sources, derived from the diet or derived from synthesis in the tissue, chiefly the liver. In the diet cholesterol comes solely from foods of animal origin (egg yolk, liver and fatty meats, cheese). Around 80% of total body cholesterol is manufactured in the liver, which means that only 15-20% of cholesterol comes from your diet. Cholesterol travels from the liver through the bloodstream to the various tissues in the body by means of a special class of protein molecules called lipoproteins. The cells take what they need, and any excess remains in the bloodstream until other lipoproteins pick it up for transport back to the liver.

Cholesterol made by the liver for tissues is transported in the largest of lipoprotein particles (very low density lipoproteins, VLDL). In the plasma, these are transformed to smaller lipoproteins (intermediate density lipoproteins, IDLP, and low density lipoproteins, LDL) by the action of enzymes. Cholesterol delivered directly to tissues is in the LDL form. Once inside the tissue cells, cholesterol is utilised for the variety of functions previously outlined. The excess cholesterol is packed in the smallest of lipoprotein particles (high density lipoprotein, HDL) and transported back to the liver for processing. For our purposes let's concentrate on the two main types of lipoproteins: LDL (about 70% of the plasma total) and HDL (about 25% of the plasma total).

LDLs are often referred to as 'bad cholesterol', HDLs as 'good cholesterol'.
It is important to recap their functions once more. Low density lipoproteins are heavily laden with cholesterol, because they are the molecules that transport cholesterol from the liver to all of the cells of the body. High density molecules on the other hand carry relatively little cholesterol, and circulate in the blood stream removing excess cholesterol from the blood and tissues. After HDLs travel through the bloodstream and collect the excess cholesterol, they return it to the liver, where it may once again be incorporated into LDLs for delivery to the cells. If everything is functioning as it should, this system remains in balance. However, if there is too much cholesterol for the HDLs to pick up promptly, or if there are not enough HDLs to do the job, cholesterol can form plaque that sticks to artery walls and may eventually cause heart disease.

It is a simple fact that persons with high HDL levels and relatively low LDL levels have a lower risk of heart disease. Even in cases where clogged arteries exist, an increase in HDL levels and a decrease in LDL levels can result in an improvement of arterial obstruction.

So what makes the LDL 'bad cholesterol' too high?

Firstly, we need to establish a set 'safe level' of both LDL and HDL combined as a total serum cholesterol reading at 200 milligrams per decilitre of blood (mg/dl). A reading above 200 indicates an increased potential for developing heart disease. A level of 200 to 239 is borderline, and those with levels over

240 are considered to be at high risk. The normal HDL range for adult men is 45 to 50 mg/dl, and that for women is 50 to 60 mg/dl. It should be noted that women, probably because of their higher oestrogen levels, have lower LDL and higher HDL contents than men, accounting for their lower incidence of arteriosclerosis. It is suggested that higher HDL levels, such as 70 or 80 mg/dl, may protect against heart disease. An HDL level under 35 mg/dl is considered risky. So if you have a cholesterol reading of 200, with HDL at 80 and LDL at 120, you are considered at low risk for heart disease. On the other hand, even if you have a total cholesterol level well under 200, you are still considered to be at increased risk of developing cardiovascular disease if your HDL level is under 35. In other words, as your HDL decreases, your potential for heart problems intensifies, even if your total is on the low side.

In the UK the cholesterol readings are often measured in units called millimoles per litre of blood, usually shortened to 'mmol/litre' or 'mmol/l'. America uses the units milligrams per decilitre of blood, mg/dl, instead. In the UK the health professional's recommendations are that it is desirable to have a total cholesterol level under 5 mmol/l, and an LDL level under 3 mmol/l.

- **ideal level:** cholesterol level in the blood less than 5mmol/l.
- **mildly high cholesterol level:** between 5 to 6.4mmol/l.
- **moderately high cholesterol level:** between 6.5 to 7.8mmol/l.
- **very high cholesterol level:** above 7.8mmol/l.

If we eat large quantities of meat and other foods containing animal products or derived from animals then high cholesterol can result. However, dietary cholesterol is only part of the story. There are other substances that affect cholesterol levels. Saturated fats, for example, have been shown to increase cholesterol levels even more than dietary cholesterol does - so even if a food product label proclaims 'No Cholesterol!' the product may still have a negative effect on your cholesterol level. Michelle Smyth of Which? says, 'You may have something which says it is low in cholesterol or low in fat and good for your heart. But, when you look at the nutritional information, it may be high in sugar or salt. This means the benefit you are being told about for the product may be counteracted by another factor and that is something people don't always realise.'

It is important to note that dietary cholesterol may or may not contribute to heart disease depending on how the individual's liver is able to regulate the plasma cholesterol level and the production of LDL. Certainly we know the body needs fats, but they must be the right kind. Good fats supply essential fatty acids, which are a very important link in our health chain. All cell membranes are composed of fats. Fats supply energy, act as an intestinal lubricant and carry the fat-soluble vitamins A, D, E, and K in the body. Unfortunately many of us in the West consume much too much of the wrong fats - that is, saturated, hydrogenated, and heated fats – which are linked to obesity, cardiovascular disease, and certain types of cancer.

Many fast-food restaurants use beef tallow (fat) to make their hamburgers, fish, chicken and French fried potatoes. Not only do these fried foods contain high amounts of cholesterol, but also this fat is subjected to high temperatures in the deep-frying process, resulting in oxidation and the formation of free radicals. Heating fat, especially frying food in fat, also produces toxic trans-fatty acids, which seem to behave much like saturated fats in clogging the arteries and raising blood cholesterol. There are other substances that raise cholesterol too. Sugar and alcohol both raise the level of natural cholesterol (that which the body produces). Although fast food chain McDonald's is not the sole culprit in marketing unhealthy foods, an article in the Daily Mail served to highlight the trans-fat problem in fast foods. The paper reported that McDonald's had revealed that its French fries contained around a third more trans-fats than it previously thought, saying it made the discovery as a result of 'enhanced testing' methods. This means that the level of trans-fat in a packet of the fast food company's large fries is 8g, up from 6g, with total fat increasing to 30g from 25g. Michael Jacobson of the US Centre for Science said, 'Nutritionally, it's a disastrous product'. However, Cathy Kapica, global nutrition director for McDonald's, said that it was 'important to note that the McDonald's menu offers choice and variety'.

Certain drugs can elevate cholesterol levels. These include steroids, oral contraceptives, furosemide (Lasix) and other diuretics, and levodopa (L-dopa, sold under the brand names Dopar, Larodopar, and Sinemet), which is used to treat Parkinson's disease. Beta-blockers, often prescribed to control high blood pressure, can cause unfavourable changes in the ratio of LDL to HDL in the blood. Cigarette smoke contains large quantities of free radicals, many known to oxidise LDL cholesterol, making them more likely to be deposited on the walls of the blood vessels. The effect of cigarette smoke may be due to the direct oxidation of lipids and proteins, and it may also have indirect effects, such as the depletion of various antioxidant defences, which then allow other cellular processes (inflammation, for example) to modify LDL. In addition, smoking increases levels of LDL, lowers levels of HDL and increases the blood's tendency to form clots. Underactive Thyroid and stress also result in an overproduction of natural cholesterol, and obesity causes unfavourable changes in serum lipoprotein levels.

Finally, one in 500 people has a genetic predisposition to high cholesterol called familial hyperlipidaemia, which prevents even the healthiest diet from lowering LDL levels. You might be interested to know about a molecule called Apolipoprotein E found in the blood. Which type you have is genetically determined. Apolipoprotein E4 contributes to blood cholesterol levels. More Finns have E4 than do Japanese, which may be one reason why the Finns have more heart disease. (1-2)

What are Triglycerides?

Triglycerides are fats carried in the blood from the food we ingest, they are carried in the bloodstream as serum-soluble lipoproteins, or lipid-carrying proteins. Triglycerides are measured as an indirect index of triglyceride-containing lipoproteins. It is said the average American ingests around

300 mg of cholesterol per day, compared with 60,000-120,000 mg (60-120 grams) of triglycerides i.e., 200 to 400 times greater than dietary cholesterol from fat intake. It means that most of the fats we eat, including butter, margarines and oils, are in triglyceride form and as the name suggests are one of three types of fats.

- Monoglycerides which are made up of one fatty acid group.
- Diglycerides which are made from two fatty acid groups,
- Triglycerides which are made up of three fatty acid groups.

Triglycerides are an efficient storage method for fats, because they take multiple fatty acid molecules and combine them with a glycerol molecule to store multiple fats in one fat molecule. For this reason, the body prefers to use triglycerides for energy storage whenever possible.

What role do Triglycerides play in the body?

They serve as a source of energy (fatty acids from triglycerides are used for muscular work or stored as body fat for future energy production). Ingested fats are either burned up immediately as fuel, or else stored in the adipose tissue where triglycerides are kept until signaled by certain hormones to be released again into the bloodstream to be used as fuel. So there is a mechanism whereby your liver will quickly convert unused calories, especially simple carbohydrates, into triglycerides for storage. So if you're eating more calories than you expend especially alcohol and sugar, your liver will most likely be storing many of those calories as triglycerides in fat cells throughout the body.

Additionally Triglycerides carry the fat-soluble vitamins A, D, E and vitamin K, an important nutrient in normal blood coagulation. They also provide thermal insulation and contribute to the structure of membranes by the formation of a lipid bilayer which has been firmly established as the universal basis for cell-membrane structure. In short Triglycerides like Cholesterol are vital for our ability to function, its only excessive amounts of both that cause health problems.

Triglyceride levels

Firstly we have to say that elevated triglycerides may be a consequence of other disease, such as untreated diabetes mellitus or nephritic syndrome or chronic renal failure. Other reasons for higher triglyceride levels tend to be, hypothyroidism, liver disease, overeating, obesity, excessive consumption of alcohol as well as rare genetic problems that impact body fat metabolism. Particular medications can also be implicated like, contraception pills, beta blockers, steroids, isotretinoin, protease inhibitors and diuretics as well as tamoxifen can all contribute to signs of enhanced elevation of triglycerides in your body.

High levels of triglycerides are strongly associated with the risk of stroke and heart disease especially in women. In a study involving postmenopausal women (aged 48 to 76 years old) conducted by a research group from the Center for Clinical and Basic Research in Ballerup, Denmark, it was found that women who had an enlarged waist and elevated levels of triglycerides had almost a five-fold increased risk of fatal cardiovascular events compared to women without those traits. The women at risk deposited fat centrally in their intra-abdominal compartment, rather than in their hips, thighs, and buttocks.

If we look at both sexes researchers accounted for other risk factors for strokes, people with more than 200 mg of triglycerides per dl of blood were nearly 30% more likely to have an ischemic stroke or TIA than people with lower levels of triglycerides.

Ischemic strokes, which occur when a blood clot or narrowed artery cuts off the brain's blood supply, account for about 80% of all strokes. The other 20% of strokes are caused by a rupture in blood vessels in the brain. High triglycerides and the low levels of HDL - the 'good' - cholesterol which usually co-exist are important risk factors for the main type of stroke - ischemic strokes - among patients with heart disease.

It is important to note that triglycerides are only really accurately measured after an 8 to 12 hour fast.

It is believed that the triglycerides/HDL ratio is one of the most potent predictors of heart disease. And that it is generally considered that if this number is below 2 the person is at a low risk of heart disease. So, the lower your triglycerides, or the higher your HDL, the smaller this ratio becomes.

Triglyceride diet

Firstly it's worth pointing out that most triglycerides hit the bloodstream 3 to 6 hours after a meal and are burned or stored within 10 to 12 hours. So the type of foods ingested will have that delayed effect but it's not straight forward just labeling fats in the diet as the only culprit as you will see.

What kind of diet will give us the right fats?

The Mediterranean Style Diet which comprises pulses, fresh fruit, wholegrains, vegetables, fish and olive oil. It is low in saturated fat but high in monosaturated fatty acids. People who follow a Mediterranean Diet tend to have higher HDL cholesterol levels and normal Triglyceride levels. The Mediterranean Diet consists of a healthy balance between omega-3 and omega-6 fatty acids.

Now we have to talk sugar

There is some very compelling research showing that carbohydrates raise triglyceride levels more significantly than fat consumption, as carbohydrates raise insulin levels. Insulin inhibits the metabolism of triglycerides in the blood to be used for energy, so high insulin levels over time can contribute to the accumulation of triglycerides.

Eating carbohydrates has the biggest effect on raised triglyceride levels and here is why – Normal fasting levels of blood glucose are in the range of 70-110mg/100 cc of blood a value that remains constant throughout life. When this level is exceeded such as after a meal rich in carbs (bread, potatoes, rice), the excess glucose in the blood is sensed by glucose detectors in the pancreas, resulting in release of insulin into the blood.

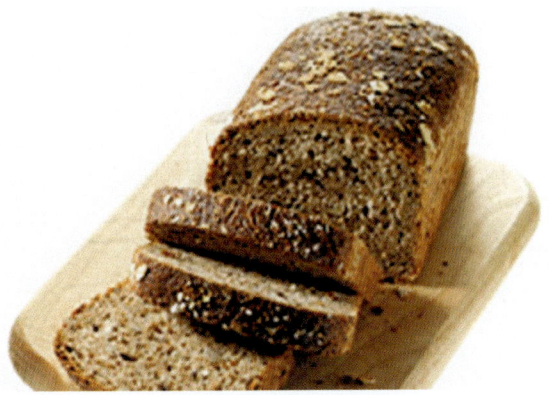

Insulin is then transported with the blood to its target tissues binding with receptors of the target cells. This binding somehow increases the permeability of the target cells to glucose, resulting in increased uptake of this substance.

Muscle cells normally prefer to use glucose for oxidation and cellular energy metabolism. But what has this got to do with my elevated Triglycerides? Now bear with me we are coming to that, you see, insulin also promotes glucose entrance into the fat cells of adipose tissue, (connective tissue which contains cells that store energy in the form of fat). Here the increased glucose supply is not utilized to provide energy for the fat cells. Instead each glucose molecule is metabolized to form two molecules of glycerol, which is used along with fatty acids to form triglycerides, the storage form of fat. In simple terms too many carbs = stored triglycerides which if you have other metabolic health factors such as obesity, high blood pressure and insulin resistance is a marker for chronic health problems.

We have mentioned glucose, in fact anything with an ose on the end is a form of sugar - sucrose, lactose, maltose, fructose, galactose…you get the idea. Something called the glycemic index will tell you how quickly a carbohydrate food breaks down into the simple sugars which are ultimately converted to glucose. Basically the higher the index number the faster the breakdown to simple sugars the more you work your pancreas to over produce insulin and so the cycle goes on.

Now you know that exceeding your body's requirements for ingesting carbohydrates is going to end up as stored triglycerides. Or to really get the point across, the donut you ate today washed down with a high fructose drink could be heading for your hips and belly tomorrow!

Now it's back to Cholesterol…..

Chapter 2

WHAT ARE THE IMPLICATIONS FOR HEALTH?

According to the British Heart Foundation statistics for 2005, high cholesterol is very common in the UK. About two out of three adults have a cholesterol level higher than is considered healthy.

- **After the age of 55, more women have high cholesterol than men.** One theory about this is that the rise in cholesterol among older women may be caused by a drop in levels of the hormone oestrogen in their bodies. Oestrogen is the main female sex hormone and is thought to help keep cholesterol down.
- **Some ethnic groups are affected more than others by high cholesterol.** Although people from certain ethnic minority groups tend to have lower total cholesterol than average, some groups - particularly Bangladeshi, Indian, Pakistani and Caribbean men - have low levels of good (HDL) cholesterol and slightly raised blood triglycerides. Researchers are not sure why this is, but it may be due to differences either in genes or in people's diets.

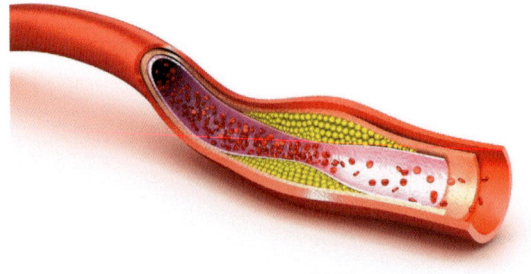

Cholesterol plays an important role in causing atherosclerosis, a specific type of arteriosclerosis (hardening of the arteries). In the West, heart disease is the number one killer responsible for nearly half of all deaths, mostly in men and in the elderly.

Cholesterol is deposited in large amounts in the victim's arterial wall. When the inner wall of an artery is damaged, platelets (important to blood clotting) adhere to the site of damage. Plasma cholesterol is deposited on these lesions, along with calcium ions, forming hard, calcified cholesterol plaques (atherosclerosis). These plaques lead to hardening of the arterial walls and loss of elasticity and responsiveness to changes in blood pressure. Plaques in the kidney may lead to chronic high blood pressure (hypertension). The plaques can cause a narrowing inside the arteries, reducing blood flow to a region where cells may experience ischaemia (oxygen starvation) due to insufficient circulation. If one of the coronary arteries becomes obstructed by accumulated deposits, or by a blood clot that has either formed or snagged on the deposit, the heart muscle will be starved for oxygen and an individual will suffer a heart attack, also referred to as a myocardial infarction (MI) or coronary occlusion (a coronary). These clots can block blood flow to a region (thrombosis). Most heart attacks and strokes are due either to atherosclerosis directly or to thrombosis caused by it. Plaques in the heart and the brain are the principle causes of heart attacks and strokes.

Heart Attack

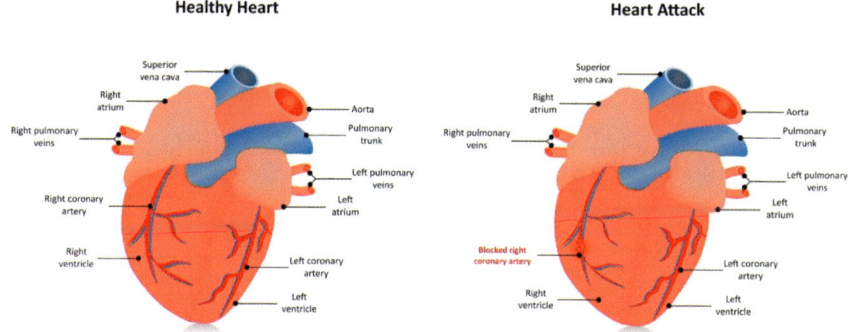

Peripheral Atherosclerosis is a disabling condition involving the extremities, which can be caused by cholesterol levels. In the early stages, the major arteries that carry blood to the legs and the feet become narrowed by fatty deposits. Atherosclerosis of the leg or foot can not only limit a person's mobility, but can also lead to loss of a limb. People who have diseased arteries in the leg or foot are likely to have them elsewhere, mainly in the heart and the brain. Early signs of peripheral atherosclerosis are aching muscles, fatigue, and cramp like pains in the ankles and legs. Depending on which arteries are blocked, there may also be pain in the hips and thighs.

Pain in the legs (often in the calf, but sometimes in the foot, thigh, hip or buttocks) that is brought on by walking and is promptly relieved by rest is called intermittent claudication. This is often the first symptom of developing peripheral atherosclerosis. Additional symptoms include numbness, weakness, and a heavy feeling in the legs. These symptoms occur because the amount of oxygenated blood that makes it through the plaque-clogged arteries is insufficient to meet the needs of the exercising leg muscles. The closer the problem lies to the abdominal aorta (the central artery that branches into the legs) the more tissue is affected and the more dangerous is the condition.

A simple test can determine how well the blood is flowing through the arteries of the legs. There are three places on the lower leg where a pulsating artery can be felt by lightly touching the skin covering the artery. One spot is the top of the foot, the second is the inner aspect of the ankle, and the third spot is behind the knee. Apply pressure lightly to the skin on these spots. If you cannot find a pulse, this is an indication that the artery supplying the leg may be narrowed. Special studies may be needed. Consult your doctor.

Chapter 3

WHAT IS THE CONVENTIONAL APPROACH TO TREATMENT?

The conventional response to raised cholesterol levels is to restrict fat in the diet and to prescribe drugs which lower these levels.

Let's examine the methodology behind the use of lipid lowering drugs which are generally prescribed only when dietary measures have failed to control hyperlipidaemia (high levels of fat in the blood). The drugs may be given at an earlier stage to individuals at increased risk of atherosclerosis - such as diabetics and people already suffering from circulatory disorders. The drugs may remove existing atheroma in the blood vessels and prevent accumulation of new deposits.

For maximum benefit these drugs are used in conjunction with a low fat diet and a reduction in other risk factors such as obesity and smoking. The choice of drug depends on the type of lipid causing problems, so a full medical history, examination, and laboratory analysis of blood samples are needed before drug treatment is prescribed.

According to the British Medical Association the following information is given regarding cholesterol and triglycerides. One or both may be raised, influencing the choice of lipid lowering drug. Bile salts contain a large amount of cholesterol and are normally released into the small intestine to aid digestion before being reabsorbed into the blood. Drugs that bind to bile salts reduce cholesterol levels by blocking their reabsorption, allowing them to be lost from the body. This action reduces the levels of bile salts in the blood, and triggers the liver to convert more cholesterol into bile salts thus reducing blood cholesterol levels.

Other drugs act on the liver. Fatty acids in the blood are normally converted into lipids by enzyme activity in the liver. Several drugs alter the way fatty acids are taken into the liver cells and others alter the enzyme activity in the liver to prevent manufacture of lipids. Fibrates and nicotinic acid and its derivatives can reduce the level of both cholesterol and triglycerides in the blood. Statins and Probucol lower blood cholesterol. It is important to note that lipid lowering drugs do not correct the underlying cause of raised levels of fat in the blood, so the doctor's advice is that it is usually necessary to continue with diet and drug treatment indefinitely. Stopping treatment usually leads to a return of high blood lipid levels.

Common Drugs

Fibrates

Bezafibrate
Ciprofibrate
Clofibrate
Fenofibrate
Gemfibrozil

Statins currently available on the US market include:

Fluvastatin (Lescol)
Pravastatin (Pravachol)
Simvastatin (Zocor)
Atorvastatin (Lipitor)
Lovastatin   (Mevacor)
Rosuvastatin (Crestor)

Drugs that bind to bile salts

Cholestyramine
Colestipol

Nicotinic acid and derivatives

Acipimox
Nicotinic Acid

Other drugs acting on the liver (Omega-3 marine triglycerides)

Probucol

What are the possible side effects of taking lipid lowering drugs?

According to the British Medical Journal, by increasing the amount of bile in the digestive tract, several drugs can cause gastrointestinal disturbances such as nausea and diarrhoea, especially at the start of treatment. In addition drugs that bind to bile salts can limit absorption of some fat-soluble vitamins, so vitamin supplements may be needed. The fibrates can increase susceptibility to gallstones and occasionally upset the balance of fats in the blood. Statins are used with caution where there is reduced liver function, and monitoring of blood samples is often advised.

Lynne McTaggart, in her book What Doctors Don't Tell You – The Truth about the Dangers of Modern Medicine, points to a number of additional side effects such as a decrease in serotonin, a brain hormone which normally keeps harmful impulses, such as aggressive behaviour and depression, in check. Californian researchers found that depression was three times more common in those with low blood cholesterol than in elderly patients over 70 with higher blood cholesterol levels. Women placed on very low-fat diets have lower levels of tryptophan, (an essential amino acid acting as a precursor of serotonin). (3) There is evidence that patients suffering from severe depression have low levels of tryptophan. (4)

Cholestyramine can cause constipation, flatulence, heartburn, nausea, diarrhoea, stomach upsets, skin rashes and, rarely, fat in the faeces. It can also lead to vitamin K deficiency, which may increase bleeding due to the inability of the blood to clot properly. In animal studies, cholestyramine has been linked with intestinal cancer. (5) Cases of sexual dysfunction have been reported in patients taking Gemfibrozil, another cholesterol lowering drug. Several studies have shown that certain cholesterol drugs may increase rates of cancer by a third. (6)

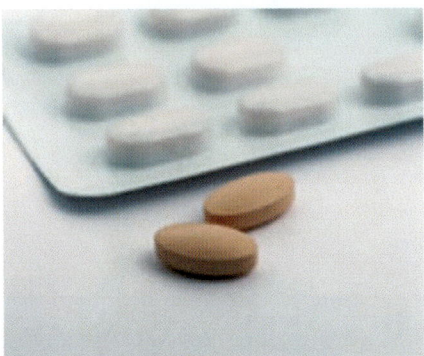

Statins - Highly popular - and highly priced - statins appeared on the market over 15 years ago to combat high cholesterol and reduce the risk of heart disease. Now millions of people around the world, with both severely and moderately high cholesterol, take one brand of statin or another. With at least 12 million Americans taking cholesterol lowering drugs, mostly statins, experts are recommending that another 23 million should be taking them.

Enthusiastic accounts of the effectiveness and safety of statins have made it the third most popular drug in the United States in terms of prescriptions filled, and the largest drug in dollar volume (Statins account for about 6.5 percent of all drug sales in the U.S., according to Forbes magazine, and earn drug companies about $26 billion per year). Pfizer's cholesterol cutting drug Lipitor was the best selling treatment for the fifth year in a row, bringing in $12.2 billion in 2005, according to data compiled by Bloomberg. Pfizer said revenue from Lipitor would exceed $13 billion in 2006.* The company plans to keep sales growing through an advertising campaign direct to consumers to convince them of the benefits of lowering cholesterol.

> * Update March 2012. Lipitor is the biggest selling drug of all time, generating sales of $106 billion over the last decade. This cholesterol-lowering drug lost patent protection on November 30th, 2011.

In March 2006, an article in the Daily Telegraph written by Celia Hall, the paper's Medical Editor, was headlined ' Heart Drug is found to turn clock back on furred arteries'. It trumpeted the results of a trial released in America which showed that the drug Rosuvastatin, when given in high doses to patients with mild heart disease, reduced the build-up of fatty deposits in arteries by up to nine per cent. Dr Neal Uren, who led the Scottish arm of the international study, said, 'For the first time we have shown that it is possible essentially to turn the clock back in the arteries of people with heart disease. This is the first time we have seen significant reversal of the fatty deposits that clog up arteries. This has exciting implications for people at risk of heart disease'. Dr Uren, a consultant cardiologist at the Edinburgh Royal Infirmary, said the good results were in line with earlier studies using weaker statins – drugs in the same class – which showed that the thickening process could be halted.

He suggested that GPs might need to be encouraged to prescribe higher doses of statins providing 'intensive' therapy. These comments represent a new use for Rosuvastatin, which is not currently licensed for atherosclerosis but is licensed for cholesterol lowering. The latest study involved 349 patients over two years. They were given 40mg of Rosuvastatin, the highest licensed dose. The drug was also found to be responsible for a 53 per cent reduction in bad cholesterol and a 15 per cent increase in good cholesterol.

Each year, nearly 260,000 people in Britain have a heart attack, of whom a third die before reaching hospital. But deaths are falling partly because of the increasing use of statins. Dr Sarah Jarvis, a London GP and member of the Royal College of General Practitioners, said the news was 'dramatically exciting' and its importance 'cannot be underestimated'.

Professor Peter Weissberg, the medical director of the British Heart Foundation, was more cautious. 'This is an important study as it is one of the first to report on the newest statin, Rosuvastatin. It uses a very aggressive approach, with the highest dose of what is the most potent statin on the market.' He added, 'This study was not designed to test whether this treatment actually saved lives. So while the results sound promising and are likely to translate into a better outcome for heart patients, we still need further studies to confirm whether these translate to fewer heart attacks.'

Let's examine the known side effects of just one type of statin called Simvastatin (brand name Zocor), remembering that this is less potent than Rosuvastatin. Simvastatin may cause the following symptoms: dry mouth, nosebleeds, increased breathlessness, and severe itching. It is stated in MIMS (Monthly Index of Medical Specialities) that adverse reactions to this drug could also include headache, asthenia (weakness or debility), abdominal pain, alopecia (loss of hair), dizziness, muscle cramps, myalgia (muscle pain), pancreatitis (inflammation of the pancreas), paraesthesia (a sensation of tingling, pricking, or numbness of the skin with no apparent physical cause), and peripheral neuropathy (a condition caused by damage to the nerves in the peripheral nervous system). The peripheral nervous system includes nerves that run from the brain and spinal cord to the rest of the body. Peripheral neuropathy is usually felt at first as tingling and numbness in the hands and feet. Symptoms can be described as burning, shooting pain, throbbing, aching, and feeling 'like frostbite' or 'walking on a bed of coals'. Further possible reactions to Simvastatin include anaemia (a deficiency of red blood cells which can lead to a lack of oxygen carrying ability, causing unusual tiredness and other symptoms) and, on rare occasions, rhabdomyolysis. Rhabdomyolysis is a disorder involving injury to the kidney resulting from the toxic effects of certain contents of muscle cells. It occurs when the iron-containing pigment myoglobin, found in the skeletal muscle, enters the bloodstream. The skeletal muscle releases myoglobin into the bloodstream after the muscle suffers damage. The kidneys attempt to filter the myoglobin out of the bloodstream, but the myoglobin can occlude the structures within the kidney, resulting in damage such as acute tubular necrosis or kidney failure. The myoglobin then may break down into additional toxic compounds, which can cause further kidney damage and failure. In addition, the dead (necrotic) skeletal muscle can cause large shifts in fluid from the bloodstream into the muscle, which reduces the relative fluid volume of the body and can lead to shock and reduced blood flow to the kidney, hepatitis (inflammation of the liver), jaundice, and myopathy (abnormal conditions or disease of the muscle tissues).

Cardiologist Peter Langsjoen notes that statin treatment may lead to heart muscle weakening and failure. (7,8) 'It occurs because statin drugs block the production of coenzyme Q10, vital for the production of cell energy,' says Langsjoen. 'Evidence to the FDA shows marked reduction of CoQ10 in patients on statin drugs.' (9)

The final point to be borne in mind is the use of long term drug therapy to lower cholesterol levels, where it is unclear what the full effects might be over a 30 year period. In spite of this, the Food and Drug Administration (FDA) gives approval for this class of drugs on the basis of less than 10 years' clinical trials.

Surgery and Other Procedures

An angiography (an X-ray examination of blood vessels) is often performed to determine whether a surgical or other procedure is necessary. In the case of atherosclerosis, this test is performed to examine blood vessels in a particular location such as the heart, brain, or lower extremities. Several different procedures (surgical and non-surgical) may be performed depending upon the location and severity of atherosclerosis.

Non-surgical techniques

The following non-operative techniques may be performed on individuals with coronary and peripheral artery disease:

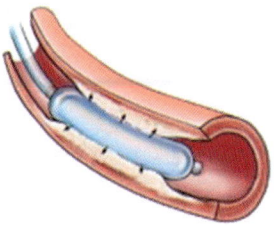

- Angioplasty—a procedure used to widen narrowed arteries. A surgeon inserts a catheter with a deflated balloon into the narrowed part of the artery. The balloon is inflated, widening the inner diameter of the blood vessel so blood can flow more easily. The balloon is then deflated and the catheter is removed. This procedure may also include the placement of a permanent stent (wire mesh) that holds the artery open and improves blood flow. Angioplasty with stent placement is considered the safest and most effective procedure for atherosclerosis.
- Atherectomy—a procedure to remove plaque from the arteries using a laser catheter or a rotating shaver.
- Laser revascularisation—a procedure in which a laser creates multiple channels through the heart muscle into the main pumping chamber of the heart. These channels fill with blood from the pumping chamber, the blood then supplying oxygen and needed nutrients to the heart muscle. The technique is used to relieve severe chest pain in individuals who have no other treatment options.

Surgical Procedures

— Bypass surgery—a procedure that reroutes or bypasses blood around clogged arteries to improve blood supply to affected areas such as the heart or the lower extremities.
— Minimally invasive bypass surgery—this procedure creates a small incision rather than the broad opening in the chest wall created during regular bypass surgery.
— Endarterectomy—a procedure primarily used to remove plaque in the carotid (a major artery located in the front of the neck) or peripheral arteries.

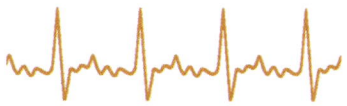

Chapter 4

WHAT ARE THE ALTERNATIVES TO CONVENTIONAL MEDICINE?

Firstly, we have to accept that until we experience a cardiovascular problem like high blood pressure or angina we probably have no idea whether we are susceptible to high cholesterol levels.
A good place to start is with the liver.

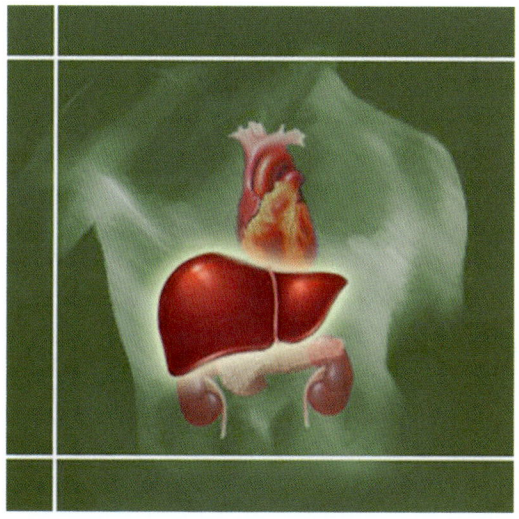

Every twenty minutes your entire blood supply goes through your liver which makes it probably the hardest working organ in the body. In addition to its normal functions of controlling the metabolism, deactivating hormones, drugs and toxins and producing bile to break down and absorb fat, a 'western liver' has to deal with up to 30,000 chemicals daily, absorbed through the skin, ingested or breathed in from the air (60 years ago this figure was just 300).

When we reach the section in this chapter concerned with the dos and don'ts of diet, it must be remembered that the liver will produce cholesterol if not enough is present. It is an important factor in maintaining good health. Therefore it is doubtful whether the efforts to lower cholesterol content by all means are justified, especially in the avoidance of foods containing cholesterol such as eggs and butter or using drugs that affect the production of cholesterol in the liver.

What are typical signs of a stressed liver?

- **Feeling nauseous at times**
- **Poor appetite**
- **Eyesight varies throughout the day**
- **'Sick' headaches (feeling down and out)**
- **High cholesterol**
- **Depression for no apparent reason**
- **Sudden outbursts of irritability**
- **Lack of motivation**
- **Overweight, especially around the middle (apple shaped people with fat concentrated around the abdomen and a waist in excess of 40 inches)**
- **Bad breath**
- **Some skin problems can be from the liver**
- **A yellow or brown coated tongue**
- **Digestive problems such as heartburn, reflux and bloating**
- **Irritable Bowel Syndrome or similar bowel problems**
- **Gall bladder problems, often associated with pain in the right shoulder blade**
- **Allergies**
- **A weak immune system**
- **Age spots, sometimes called 'liver spots'**

Any sensible course to detoxify and fortify the liver must begin by dealing with any bowel conditions such as constipation, irritable bowel, diverticulitis or colitis. A person's psychological state and behaviour can also have a direct effect on the liver through conditions such as stress, anxiety, frustration and especially anger. A great maxim in life comes from my late uncle Bert who said, 'Look not back in anger nor forward in fear but around in awareness'.

There are a number of supplements which help to support a healthy liver and circulatory system, including:

Lecithin (the name lecithin is derived from the Greek word for egg yolk), in the presence of quality oils such as cold pressed safflower or sunflower seed oil, helps break down residual fats in the liver. Because eggs contain both lecithin and cholesterol it runs counter to the conventional advice not to eat free range or organic eggs if you are an atherosclerotic patient. In the Green Library information sheet N022 the following advice is given: 'For an adult, the recommended granular lecithin intake is 2 heaped tablespoons together with a tablespoon of cold pressed safflower oil or sunflower oil. These may be taken mixed in a fruit juice of choice, or with breakfast cereal, mixed with yoghurt or simply sprinkle the granular lecithin on a salad and use this excellent oil as a base for the salad dressing. In addition a daily intake of vitamin C, vitamin E and a good quality multivitamin-mineral supplement can combine to help in dissolution of cholesterol plaques in the arteries. Cholesterol and lecithin need to combine in the presence of adequate linoleate (safflower has a particularly high content). When they do, there is a lowering of the melting point of cholesterol below body temperature. Without the availability of the oil, cholesterol has a very high melting point and may form insoluble plaques in the arterial walls. It is claimed that by using lecithin in this way, atherosclerosis in the less advanced cases where the arteries have not lost their flexibility is reversible over a period of months.'

Finally, lecithin is an important component of bile, aiding emulsification of dietary fats and providing essential fatty acids. Lecithin is a rich source of choline which the liver converts to phosphatidylcholine, a precursor of acetylcholine which is a neurotransmitter. It helps the brain to function better and maintains good memory functions.

Milk Thistle, also commonly known as silymarin, is a well known traditional herb that has been used for many years in Germany. Milk thistle contains some of the most potent liver-protecting substances known. Prevents free radical damage by acting as an antioxidant, protecting the liver. Also stimulates the production of new liver cells and has even been shown to reverse fatty degeneration of the liver. The silybin component of silymarin has been related to cholesterol lowering effects. Protects the kidneys. Prevents formation of damaging leukotrienes, (products of arachidonic acid metabolism serving as mediators of inflammation and roles in allergic reactions). Through the capability to increase bile solubility, silymarin may also help prevent or alleviate gallstones. Good for adrenal disorders, inflammatory bowel disorders, weakened immune system, and all liver disorders such as jaundice and hepatitis.

Dandelion cleanses the bloodstream and liver, and increases the production of bile. Also reduces serum cholesterol and uric acid. Improves functioning of the kidneys, pancreas, spleen, and stomach. Useful for cirrhosis of the liver, fluid retention, hepatitis, jaundice and may aid in prevention of age spots.

Artichoke lowers blood cholesterol, acts as a diuretic and liver tonic, and lowers blood sugar. It protects the liver against toxins and infection and in addition it stimulates regeneration of liver cells. The following effects on the liver have been demonstrated:

- Promotion of blood circulation
- Mobilisation of energy reserves
- Increase in the number of hepatocytes with double nuclei
- Increase in the RNA content of liver cells
- Stimulation of cell division.

Clinical trials on 84 patients with secondary hyperlipidaemia were performed using artichoke. The following lipid values in serum were tested: total cholesterol, LDL cholesterol, HDL cholesterol, and triglycerides. Though there was a dramatic increase in HDL cholesterol, artichoke caused a decrease in value of the other parameters. (10)

Berberis (also known as Barberry) is one of the best remedies for correcting liver function and promoting the flow of bile. Its use is indicated when there is an inflammation of the gall bladder or in the presence of gallstones, also when jaundice occurs because of a congested state of the liver.

Bupleurum (Chai Hu – Hare's Ear) is first mentioned medically by the Chinese about 200AD. Because of its yellow flowers, the ancient Doctrine of Signatures assigned it to the treatment of liver and gall bladder problems. It has many helpful qualities to herbalists including its use for hepatitis, jaundice, and skin disorders.

Schizandra (Wu wei tzu) During the early 1980s, Chinese doctors began researching Schizandra as a possible treatment for hepatitis, based on its potential for liver-protective effects and the nature of its active constituents. Western herbalists commonly recommend Schizandra as support for the lungs, liver and kidneys. **CAUTION**: Schizandra should not be used during pregnancy except under medical supervision because it promotes uterine contractions during labour. Schizandra should be avoided by persons with peptic ulcers, epilepsy and high blood pressure.

Apple Pectin (Malus sylvestris) in the diets of humans and lab animals has been shown to increase the excretion of lipids, cholesterol and bile acids, and reduce serum cholesterol levels. Pectins operate by binding with bile acids, thereby decreasing cholesterol and fat absorption. Researchers at the University of California found that apple pectin also acts as an antioxidant against the damaging portion of cholesterol in the blood stream.

Citrus Pectin is a plant fibre obtained from the rind and peel of citrus fruits such as lemons, grapefruits, oranges and tangerines. Structurally, pectin is classified as a complex polysaccharide (long-chain carbohydrate) characterised by its numerous long complex side chains. At a molecular level, pectin is a strong binding agent, which directly relates to its tremendous cholesterol lowering and detoxification properties. Because of the large size and molecular weight of pectin molecules, however, its actions are limited to its activity in the digestive tract.

Red Yeast Rice has been used in traditional Chinese medicine for thousands of years as a treatment for 'bad blood'. It is made by fermenting red yeast (Monascus purpureus) on rice. Its active ingredient mevinolin is chemically identical to the cholesterol lowering compound lovostatin, and also similar to the two cholesterol lowering drugs Zocor (simvastatin) and Lipitor (atorvastatin). According to available research, red yeast rice consistently lowers total cholesterol (by an average of 10-30%), lowers LDL cholesterol (by an average of 10-20%), lowers triglycerides (by an average of 15-25%) and increases HDL cholesterol (by an average of 7-15%). It appears to accomplish this by reducing the liver's production of cholesterol.
* Caution Red Yeast Rice is a statin drug, albeit in a natural form and at a lower dosage.

Policosanol is isolated and refined from sugarcane. The active ingredient is octacosanol. Clinical studies have demonstrated policosanol has anti-inflammatory, anti-viral and neural-protective properties. Policosanol has been shown in studies to normalise cholesterol as well or better than statin drugs.

More Herbs in brief to help the liver:

Dong Quai Usually associated with female complaints this versatile herb also helps to clear liver stagnation (of both energy and toxins) and can relieve constipation, especially in the elderly. Animal studies suggest that dong quai may treat abnormal heart rhythm, prevent accumulation of platelets in blood vessels (contributing to plaque formation or atherosclerosis), protect the liver, promote urination, fight infection and promote sleep.

Goldenseal promotes functioning capacity of the colon, liver, pancreas, spleen, and lymphatic and respiratory systems.

Black Radish activates the liver cells, maintains a healthy gall bladder, aids digestion, facilitates a diuretic effect, is cleansing, is antibacterial, and can assist hepatic colic by stimulating the secretion of bile.

Red Clover Amongst many actions and uses acts as a blood purifier, is used for inflammatory bowel disorders, kidney problems and liver disease.

Yellow Dock acts as a blood purifier and cleanser, and tones the entire system. Improves colon and liver function. Good for anaemia, liver disease, and skin disorders such as eczema, hives, psoriasis, and rashes.

Raspberry Extract provides ellagic acid reported to help the liver function as well as providing biologically active antioxidant benefit.

Fo Ti (He Shou Wu) There is evidence that Fo-Ti can lower serum cholesterol, decrease hardening of the arteries, and improve immune function. There are no controlled studies on the effectiveness or safety of Fo-Ti in humans. Preliminary studies with animals have found that Fo-Ti may attenuate diet-induced increases in plasma cholesterol, LDL cholesterol, and plasma triglycerides.

Coleus Forskohlii plant is a perennial member of the mint or Lamiaceae family that was first discovered in the lower elevations of India. The root is used for a myriad of purposes including cholesterol control. The active extract is Forskohlin and has been shown to increase serum levels of HDL and significantly decrease the total cholesterol/HDL ratio.

Introducing four medicinal mushrooms with known cholesterol lowering effects.

Reishi (Ganoderma lucidum)

Called "Mushroom of Immortality" Reishi is known as Lingzhi in China, or "spirit plant." Reishi has been used medicinally in Asia for thousands of years. In addition to its antiviral, antibacterial antifungal and anti-inflammatory it has been shown to normalize blood cholesterol levels and blood pressure.

Shiitake (Lentinula edodes)

Shiitake is a popular culinary mushroom used in dishes around the world. It contains a number of health-stimulating agents, including lentinan, the polysaccharide for which it was named. Lentinan has been isolated and used to treat stomach and other cancers due to its antitumor properties, but has also been found to protect your liver, relieve other stomach ailments (hyperacidity, gallstones, and ulcers), anemia, ascites, and pleural effusion.

Shiitake mushrooms also demonstrate antiviral (including HIV, hepatitis, and the "common cold"), antibacterial, and antifungal effects; blood sugar stabilization; reduced platelet aggregation; and reduced atherosclerosis. Shiitake also contains eritadenine, which has strong cholesterol-lowering properties.

Cordyceps (Cordyceps militaris)

Cordyceps, also called caterpillar fungus or Tochukasu, is a favorite of athletes because it increases ATP production, strength and endurance, and has anti-aging effects. This parasitic mushroom is unique because, in the wild, it grows out of an insect host instead of a plant host. Cordyceps has an enduring history in both traditional Chinese and Tibetan medicine. Cordyceps has hypoglycemic and possible antidepressant effects, protects your liver and kidneys, increases blood flow, helps normalize your cholesterol levels, and has been used to treat Hepatitis B. It has antitumor properties as well.

Himematsutake (Agaricus blazei)

Last but not least is mushroom Himematsutake, also called Royal Sun Agaricus, a relative of the common button mushroom. Himematsutake was not cultivated in the East until fairly recently but is now a very popular natural medicine, used by almost a half million Japanese.

Himematsutake mushroom is attracting many scientists worldwide due to its remarkable anticancer properties related to six special polysaccharides. Like many other medicinal mushrooms, this fungus can also protect you from the damaging effects of radiation and chemotherapy. But equally important are its benefits concerning observed decreases in insulin resistance in diabetics and normalization of cholesterol.

Finally for now, in the US you can buy a special type of fibre called PGX. This powder is created by reacting glucomannan a soluble fibre with other plant fibres (alginate from seaweed and xanthan gum). PGX has been shown to be very effective for losing weight. In one study over-weight volunteers lost on average 13lbs (6kg), and five inches (12cms) off their waist in a 14 week trial, while their total cholesterol dropped by almost 20 per cent, with the 'bad' LDL cholesterol dropping by a fifth.

Natural ways to maintain healthy heart function and important markers for heart health

Plant Sterols are being utilised in many countries for their cholesterol lowering properties - these natural plant fats, which are structurally very similar to cholesterol, an animal steroid, reduce absorption by competing with cholesterol for space in the mixed micelles of fats that are absorbed in the gut mucosal cells.

Vegetarians naturally consume twice the average intake of plant sterols as these molecules are prevalent in pulses, peas, vegetables, nuts, seeds and vegetable oils – too little to affect cholesterol levels. Advances in food technology, however, have produced a variety of sterols that can be cheaply produced from wood and soya and added to refined foods – notably fats – to bring daily consumption up to an effective 1g a day level. These sterols have safety approvals from the European Union's novel foods committee and the American FDA now allows products containing plant sterols to make label claims that they help reduce the risk of coronary heart disease.

Blood cholesterol levels, particularly LDL cholesterol, have been controlled by the use of sterols for over 50 years. Reductions of up to 13% in plasma LDL levels have been noted when sterols have been added to the diet.

There is concern that plant sterols may interfere with absorption of fat soluble vitamins but vitamin A, D and K uptake appears to be unaffected. Beta-carotene and vitamin E uptake may be marginally reduced but still within a normal range and a diet rich in carotenoids, found in spinach, carrots, peppers and in vitamin E, high in nuts, seeds and wholegrains, would counter any slight reductions in these fat-soluble nutrients.

Methyl Donors As more and more studies question the idea that high cholesterol is the predominant cause of heart disease, researchers are giving more attention to other risk factors such as homocysteine, fibrinogen and lipoprotein (a) levels.

Homocysteine in particular is known to be associated with pathological changes in the lining of the arteries, with negative effects on blood clotting and also with oxidation of LDL cholesterol – leading to the formation of plaque. As a result some researchers suggest it has a much more fundamental role in atherosclerosis than cholesterol, and indeed high levels lead to atherosclerosis even when cholesterol levels are 'normal'.

Important homocysteine moderators are the methyl donors B6, B12, Folate and TMG (trimethylglycine, also known as anhydrous betaine). Methyl donors are able to transfer a methyl group – a carbon atom attached to three hydrogen atoms (CH3) – to another substance in the process known as methylation. The metabolism of lipids and of DNA are among the biochemical reactions dependent on methylation. The body's powers of methylation are thought to decline with age, but this is most likely to be a result of poor nutrition. The body does not manufacture methyl groups – they must be provided in the diet and can be inhibited by imbalanced intake of lipids and by other dietary factors.

TMG is found in a variety of plant and animal sources and is perhaps the most effective methyl donor as it contains three methyl groups that can be used to convert the potentially harmful homocysteine to the beneficial amino acid methionine and subsequently produce raised levels of the protective S-adenosylmethionine (SAM-e).

Probiotics Lactic acid bacteria positively affect blood pressure and fibrinogen levels as well as having beneficial effects on LDL cholesterol levels. Lactobacillus plantarum in particular may help prevent atherosclerosis formation. Lactic acid bacteria ferment fibre in the large intestine and produce SCFAs (short chain fatty acids) including acetic, proprionic and butyric acids. Acetic and proprionic acids are absorbed into the bloodstream and become metabolised via the liver. Researchers have suggested these SCFAs improve glucose tolerance and inhibit cholesterol synthesis in the liver.

Butyric acid is also utilised by the heart muscle as oxidative fuel especially when oxygen flow to the heart is restricted, which may be the case if the coronary artery is occluded by plaque or constricted.

Due to its production of proprionic acid, supplementation of L.plantarum can also reduce inflammation and oxidative damage to LDL in the artery wall. Certain Non Steroidal Anti Inflammatory (NSAID) medications such as Ibuprofen are derivatives of proprionic acid.

In common with other lactic acid bacteria, L.plantarum is able to deconjugate bile acids in the duodenum. Bile acids are water-soluble end products of cholesterol manufactured by the liver to aid with lipid digestion. During digestion, a high proportion of the bile acids are usually returned to the liver. However, if they are broken down by a resident population of lactic acid bacteria including L.plantarum then the liver has to synthesise new bile acids from serum cholesterol. This results in a reduction in the serum levels of cholesterol and less cholesterol is available to attach to rough areas in damaged artery walls, which would become foamed by the immune system in an attempt to quell the subsequent inflammation.

C-Reactive Protein

A useful inflammation marker is the C-Reactive Protein (CRP) test. This is a substance produced by the body when arteries become inflamed and is a more powerful predictor of a person's risk of a heart attack or stroke than LDL cholesterol. It is fair to say the test is not infallible as it can sometimes point to inflammation caused by other factors such as arthritis, cancer or acute infection etc. Nonetheless there are many researchers who consider atherosclerosis as an inflammatory condition similar to other degenerative diseases. Some immunologists are even categorizing atherosclerosis as a benign tumour.

As previously stated hardening and narrowing of the arterial wall is a cumulative result of microscopic trauma with inflammation occurring in the presence of oxidized lipids. An exciting discovery of a proteolytic enzyme originating from Silkworms-Serrapeptase has been used by doctors in Europe and Asia for over 30 years to help digest atherosclerotic plaque without harming the healthy cells lining the arterial wall. This enzyme is manufactured commercially today through fermentation but was originally found in the intestine of the Silkworm. The Silkworm uses the enzyme to instantly dissolve the hard cocoon to allow the moth to escape and fly away. Serrapeptase has been shown to digest non-living tissue, blood clots, cysts, arterial plaque and inflammation in all forms. (see page 97 for more information on Serrapeptase)

Leptin in Obesity and Heart Disease

Leptin, a hormone produced by fat cells, increases with obesity and appears to play a role in the vascular complications associated with overweight conditions. Discovered in the last decade assessing leptin levels has emerged as a means of screening for heart disease.

The journal Circulation showed that men with established heart disease had blood leptin levels 16% higher than men considered heart healthy. Every 30% increase in leptin increased the risk of a heart attack or a vascular event by 25% (Wallace et al 2001). The levels of leptin, structurally a cytokine, (a category of signalling molecules that are used extensively in cellular communication.), rise in tandem with C-Reactive Protein, (CRP). These findings imply that body fat influences CRP levels (Mercola 2002a) in addition to a myriad of other health problems.

Since leptin levels correlate well with adiposity, strategies aimed at weight reduction should remain the first line of defence.

Antioxidants

Why do Eskimos, who typically eat a diet loaded with animal fat, have very low rates of heart disease?

The answer is that high cholesterol isn't the cause of heart disease - ***oxidised*** cholesterol is.

That's the opinion of many alternative physicians including Philip Lee Miller MD, founder and director of the Los Gatos Longevity Institute in California. 'I'm one of those people who have been saying for 30 years that cholesterol does not cause heart disease,' he says. 'It's a recruit in the process, like a soldier is a recruit in a war, but it does not cause the war.'

Dr Miller, like the majority of medical professionals, recognises that the lowering of LDL cholesterol plays a critical role in preventing hardening of the arteries. He knows that excess cholesterol in the bloodstream can be subjected to oxidation (the same oxygen-sparked, cell destroying process that rusts iron or turns an apple brown after it has been cut).

The destructive process of oxidation is literally inflammatory - it's like a fire in the body.

'The immune system, your body's fire service, rushes foam cells to the area to douse the blaze. But just as firemen sometimes have to axe down a door to get into a burning building, the anti-inflammatory process can damage the lining of the artery. This roughened, injured area is a perfect foundation for the build-up of plaque, the truly evil plug that clogs arteries and triggers heart attacks'.

'Oxidized LDL starts an inflammatory reaction that the body tries to heal, but the healing causes more problems than it resolves, ' says Dr Miller. The best way to prevent this heart-hurting process, he says, is to prevent the oxidation of LDL cholesterol - and the best way to do that, he adds, is to make sure you get enough of the antioxidants vitamin E, vitamin C, and glutathione.

Antioxidants work by calming unstable oxygen molecules called free radicals, which are responsible for oxidising cells. When antioxidants neutralise free radicals, they are on a type of suicide mission. The antioxidants themselves are oxidised or, in chemical terms, reduced.

Fortunately, the body has a system to help ensure that there are always plenty of antioxidants available, Dr Miller says. When vitamin C is oxidised, vitamin E comes to the rescue, donating some of its molecules to restore the vitamin C to its full antioxidant status. In the process, the vitamin E is reduced, but the glutathione replenishes it. That's why you need all three nutrients, says Dr Miller.

Vitamin C – The first line of defence against Heart Disease

Vitamin C is a very powerful antioxidant. Dr Miller recommends taking anywhere from 1,000 to 4,000 milligrams a day to reduce the oxidation of LDL and prevent heart disease.

At this point I would like to refer to the work of Drs Rath and Pauling and their breakthrough research which, in addition to recognising the antioxidant role of vitamin C, was to reveal that atherosclerosis is not a disease, but possibly the body's way of repairing or bolstering weak or damaged arteries. It was Dr Rath who was part of a group of researchers who had discovered that the major culprit in cholesterol was lipoprotein (a) [Lp(a)], an especially 'sticky' molecule that incorporates itself into the collagen found in artery walls, thereby causing atherosclerosis.

The next great insight was that animals do not get atherosclerosis – a fact well known to vets for the past 50 years. Animals produce an enzyme that converts glucose into vitamin C in the liver. Could it be that we humans are suffering from a form of scurvy caused by insufficient amounts of vitamin C which in turn forces the body to use lipoproteins in cholesterol to repair damaged arteries? Thus, atherosclerosis in humans and guinea pigs (guinea pigs and humans need vitamin C in their diet whereas all other mammalian species make their own) is due to vitamin C deficiency. The body reservoir of vitamin C in people is on average 10 to 100 times lower than the vitamin C levels in animals.

As Dr Rath reports, vitamin C is essential for the production of collagen and elastin, the elastic, fibrous materials which knit the walls of arteries and blood vessels together. Collagen cells form the structure for arteries, organs and skin, and so a chronic vitamin C deficiency causes the beginning of a collapse in the arterial walls, necessitating a healing process to commence in the form of lipoprotein (a) fats which the body attempts to use to bond the thousands of tiny breaches in the arterial walls. It is a fact that atherosclerosis mainly occurs in the vessels near the heart due to the constant mechanical stress caused by the heart's pumping force. The need for ongoing repairs of these leaky artery walls produces an overcompensation of repair materials which, in the absence of sufficient quantities of vitamin C, vitamin E, proline and lysine (amino acids), will lead to atherosclerotic deposits in the arterial walls to cover the breaches caused by the disintegrating collagen. For further information on this subject I recommend you read Dr Matthias Rath's book entitled Why Animals Don't Get Heart Attacks – But People Do! (MR Publishing).

Sources

Vitamin C is found in berries, citrus fruits, and green vegetables. Good sources include asparagus, avocados, beet greens, blackcurrants, broccoli, Brussels sprouts, cantaloupe, collards, dulse, grapefruit, kale, lemons, mangoes, onions, oranges, papayas, green peas, sweet peppers, pineapple, radishes, rose hips, spinach, strawberries, tomatoes, and watercress.

* Smokers please be aware that each cigarette destroys 25 mg of Vitamin C.

Vitamin E

Like vitamin C, vitamin E is a powerful antioxidant. Dr Miller says that 800 international units daily is the ideal dose to prevent cholesterol from oxidizing. Since cell membranes are composed of lipids, it effectively prevents the cells' protective coatings from becoming rancid as a result of the assault of free radicals. He recommends using vitamin E supplements that are natural, not synthetic. For maximum potency, they should contain mixed tocopherols: the label will specify the ingredients alpha-, beta-, and gamma-tocopherol.

'A mix of tocopherols, not just one, is the way vitamin E is found in nature,' he explains. It is to be noted that selenium enhances vitamin E uptake. These two nutrients should be taken together.

Sources

Vitamin E is found in the following food sources: cold-pressed vegetable oils, dark green leafy vegetables, legumes, nuts, seeds, and wholegrains. Significant quantities of this vitamin are also found in brown rice, cornmeal, organ meats, soybeans, sweet potatoes, watercress, wheat and wheat germ.

N-Acetylcysteine (NAC) to create Glutathione

Vitamins C and E are most effective when your body has high levels of glutathione, says Dr Miller. A doctor can measure your glutathione levels and, if they are low, Dr Miller recommends taking a supplement called NAC, which builds and conserves your body's store of glutathione.

The body does not do a good job of absorbing most glutathione supplements, Dr Miller says. But NAC, a form of the amino acid cysteine, he says, provides the right chemical precursors for your body to create glutathione. He recommends taking 3,000 milligrams a day.

Coenzyme Q10 (CoQ10)

Doctors in Japan, Sweden, Italy, and Canada commonly prescribe CoQ10 to heart patients. Research has shown that people with cardiovascular disease have low levels of CoQ10 in their hearts.

One study found that people who receive daily CoQ10 supplements within 3 days of a heart attack were significantly less likely to experience subsequent heart attacks and chest pain and were also less likely to die of the condition than those who did not receive the supplements. Acting in conjunction with enzymes (hence the name 'coenzyme'), the compound speeds up the metabolic process, providing energy that cells need to digest food, heal wounds, and maintain healthy muscles. It performs countless further bodily functions.

CoQ10 is a natural antioxidant which is reduced by the use of statins. 30-90mgs may be taken per day as a supplement. A relatively new form of coenzyme Q10 – ubiquinol – has been found to significantly lower blood levels of a form of cholesterol strongly associated with cardiovascular risk. Ubiquinol, a vitamin like substance, is also known as "reduced CoQ10" meaning that it contains a balanced set of electrons. Some research suggests that it has greater potency than the common form of CoQ10, which is known as ubiquinone.

Constance Schmeizer from the Christian Albrechts University of Kiel Germany and her colleagues asked 53 healthy men to take 150mg of ubiquinol daily for two weeks. After taking the supplements, the men's blood levels of CoQ10 increased by almost five times.

During this time, the men's LDL levels decreased by an average of 12.7 per cent. Significantly, their pattern B LDL declined by 33 per cent. High levels of pattern B LDL, which consists of tiny particles that infiltrate blood vessel walls, are regarded as the most accurate predictor of cardiovascular risk. In contrast, the ubiquinol had no effect on pattern A LDL, which consists of light and fluffy particles that do not harm blood vessel walls. In addition, the ubiquinol decreased the activity of several proinflammatory molecules called cytokines.

Sources
Mackerel, salmon, and sardines contain the largest amounts of CoQ10. It is also found in beef, peanuts, and spinach.

Vitamin A and Beta-Carotene
Vitamin A and its precursor, beta-carotene, are powerful free radical scavengers. Its intake lowers cardiovascular risk over 30%, documented in more than 87,000 study participants over six years. (11)

Sources

Vitamin A can be found in animal livers, fish liver oils, and green and yellow fruits and vegetables. Foods that contain significant amounts include apricots, asparagus, beet greens, broccoli, cantaloupe, carrots, collards, dulse, fish liver and fish liver oil, garlic, kale, papayas, peaches, pumpkin, red peppers, spirulina, sweet potatoes, spinach, turnip greens, watercress, and yellow squash.

Lycopene

This is an unsaturated carotenoid pigment which imparts the red colour in fruits and vegetables and is similar in composition to beta-carotene. Lycopene is more readily absorbed from the intestinal tract as a micelle (microcell) in the presence of mono- unsaturated oils such as olive oil as found traditionally in the Mediterranean diet.

Lycopene also protects the fatty cholesterol particles and exerts an antioxidant and anti-inflammatory effect on plaque deposits. A high lycopene intake (over 20mg a day) has been linked to a 47% reduction in heart attacks. (12)

Green Tea contains vitamins and minerals, but the primary constituents of interest are the polyphenols, particularly the catechin epigallocatechin (EGCG). Polyphenols have antioxidant potential and help maintain the activity of antioxidant enzymes such as glutathione peroxidase.

Selenium

Low blood levels of this antioxidant may worsen atherosclerosis. Cigarette smoking and alcohol ingestion are believed to contribute to selenium deficiency. This trace mineral is very helpful for controlling cholesterol. Firstly, it boosts levels of glutathione. Secondly, it works on its own to lower LDL. Thirdly, it increases healthful HDL, says Dr Miller. 'Selenium is absolutely critical to any cholesterol-lowering program,' he says. He recommends long term use of a daily multivitamin/mineral complex containing at least 200 micrograms of selenium.

Sources

Selenium can be found in meats and grains, depending on the selenium content of the soil where the food is raised. Because New Zealand soils are low in selenium, cattle and sheep raised there have suffered a breakdown of muscle tissue, including the heart muscle. However, human intake of selenium there is adequate because of imported Australian wheat. The soil of much of America farmland is low in selenium, resulting in selenium-deficient produce.

Selenium can be found in Brazil nuts, brewer's yeast, broccoli, brown rice, chicken, dairy products, dulse, garlic, kelp, liver, molasses, onions, salmon, seafood, torula yeast, tuna, vegetables, wheat germ and whole grains.

Flavonoids

Test tube, animal, and some population-based studies suggest that the flavonoids quercetin, resveratrol, and catechins (all found in high concentrations in red wine) may help reduce the risk of atherosclerosis. By acting as antioxidants, their nutrients appear to protect against the damage caused by LDL cholesterol. When choosing wines, generally go for the deepest red colour and a good tannic structure. A guide is as follows:

- **High**: Merlot, Cabernet, Sauvignon, and Chianti
- **Intermediate**: Rioja, Pinot Noir
- **Low**: Côtes du Rhône, Beaujolais, most rosé wines, whites

Oligomeric Proanthocyanidins (OPCs)

These are naturally occurring substances present in a variety of food and botanical sources. They are unique flavonols that have powerful antioxidant capabilities and excellent bioavailability. Clinical tests suggest that OPCs may be as much as fifty times more potent than vitamin E and twenty times more potent than vitamin C in terms of bioavailable antioxidant activity. In addition to their antioxidant activity, they strengthen and repair connective tissue, including that of the cardiovascular system, and they moderate allergic and inflammatory responses by reducing histamine production.

OPCs are found throughout plant life, but the two main sources are pine bark extract (Pycnogenol) and grape seed extract. Pycnogenol was the first source of OPCs discovered, and the process for extracting it was patented in the 1950s. As a result, even though Pycnogenol is a trademarked name for pine bark extract, the term is often used informally to refer to other OPC sources as well, most notably grape seed extract.

Superoxide Dismutase

Superoxide dismutase (SOD) is an enzyme. SOD revitalises cells and reduces the rate of cell destruction. It neutralises the most common and possibly the most dangerous free radical 'superoxide'. It also aids in the body's utilisation of zinc*, copper*, and manganese. There are two types of SOD: copper/zinc SOD (Cu/Zn SOD) and manganese SOD (Mn SOD). Each of these enzymes works to protect a particular part of the cell. SOD occurs naturally in barley grass, broccoli, Brussels sprouts, cabbage, wheatgrass, and most green plants.

* In the context of cholesterol, zinc and copper increase HDL and reduce LDL, says Amy Rothenberg ND, a naturopathic doctor in Enfield, Connecticut. She recommends taking 30 milligrams of zinc and 1 to 2 milligrams of copper daily, preferably as part of a multivitamin/mineral supplement. Zinc has antioxidant properties of its own and in addition is also needed for proper maintenance of vitamin E levels in the blood and aid in the absorption of vitamin A.

Melatonin

Among the newest antioxidants to be discovered, the hormone melatonin may also be the most efficient free radical scavenger that has thus far been identified. While most antioxidants work only in certain parts of certain cells, melatonin can permeate any cell in any part of the body. Melatonin also stimulates the antioxidant enzyme glutathione peroxidase. It has been noted that low levels of melatonin in the blood have been associated with heart disease, but it is not clear whether melatonin levels are low in response to heart disease or whether low levels of melatonin predispose people to developing this condition.

Hawthorn (Crataegus Monogyna)

Hawthorn has been used traditionally as a remedy for cardiovascular diseases. Studies demonstrate that this herb has antioxidant properties that help protect against the formation of plaques and may help control high cholesterol and high blood pressure.

Alpha Lipoic Acid (ALA)

Is an antioxidant compound with reported benefits in lowering triglycerides. According to Regis Moreau and colleagues at Oregon State University's Linus Pauling Institute their study with rats showed the benefit of ALA on triglyceride levels was comparable to that of currently used drugs, (the mode of action was determined to differ from fibrates).

Sources

Alpha lipoic acid is made by the body and can be found in very small amounts in foods such as spinach, broccoli, peas, Brewer's yeast, brussel sprouts, rice bran, and organ meats.

Foods for Cholesterol Control √

Many different types of foods and components of foods can help lower LDL and boost HDL. Here are the ones that health practitioners recommend most.

Apples

"I consider apples a magic food," said Bahram H. Arjmandi, Ph.D., director for the Center for Advancing Exercise and Nutrition Research on Aging at Florida State University. "Apples are not my favorite food, but I buy a bag a week and try to eat two per day. I am convinced this is what I should do if I want to remain healthy."

According to Arjmandi, apple pectin -the white stuff under the skin - binds to cholesterol in the gut and ferries it out of the body. This is well-known, but what surprised Arjmandi is how much cholesterol a couple of apples can remove from the body. In one recent study, he divided 160 women between the ages of 45 and 65 into two groups. One group ate 75 grams of dried apple per day about 2 1/2 ounces while the other ate the same amount of dried prunes. To his amazement, the women who ate apples experienced a 23 percent decrease in LDL "bad" cholesterol, and increased their HDL "good" cholesterol by 3 percent to 4 percent a boost difficult to achieve with drugs or exercise.

The women who ate the dried prunes experienced no such effects on their cholesterol. So try eating two apples a day to reduce LDL cholesterol effectively and you not only don't harm your liver (like you could with Statin therapy), but you substantially benefit your health."

Oat Bran

Oat bran is rich in beta-glucans a type of soluble fibre , a substance that binds with cholesterol in the intestine and ushers it out of the body. Dr Rothenberg recommends eating ¾ of a cup of cooked oat bran cereal a day: this, she says, can lower cholesterol by 10 per cent. The best soluble fibre by far is glucomannan from the Japanese konjac plant, it has the same actions as oat bran eliminating cholesterol by binding to it in the digestive tract and stabilizing blood sugar which is associated with improving insulin sensitivity.

Cayenne helps regulate cholesterol and lipid levels.

Turmeric a yellow coloured powder used as a food colouring agent and as a spice has been shown to exhibit favourable effects on lowering LDL Cholesterol. Research from Penn State released in March 2012 finds the spice turmeric may do the heart good by lower triglyceride and insulin levels. "Elevated triglycerides are a risk factor for heart disease," explains researcher Sheila West.

Her study concluded that incorporating turmeric in an otherwise high fat meal actually lowered triglycerides and insulin levels. Levels dropped by about one third for those using turmeric in the meal. "It was surprising," West says. "I didn't expect such a large decrease."

"To me, the biggest advantage (found in the study) is the lowering of triglycerides and the insulin levels (which dropped about 20 percent)," explains cardiologist Ravi Dave of the University of California, Los Angeles.

Cinnamon may have potential for lowering LDL Cholesterol in addition to its known properties of lowering blood sugar levels in type II diabetics. Research is continuing to determine which form of Cinnamon may be the most beneficial.

Fenugreek Seed in the diet has been shown to reduce blood glucose and plasma cholesterol levels.

Plaintain Seed has been shown by scientists in Italy, Russia and other countries to reduce the intestinal absorption of lipids.

Cilantro or Coriander

One of the oldest known spices in the world, dating back nearly 7,000 years. Contains large amounts of quercetin an antioxidant flavonoid which helps prevent LDL oxidation and protects damage to artery walls. It also shows promise in helping reduce high blood pressure that occurs as a result of artery narrowing.

Walnuts

Walnuts contain alpha-linolenic acid, which can help lower total cholesterol levels and improve the HDL/LDL cholesterol ratio. A study has found that eating walnuts at the end of a meal may help to reduce the damage fatty foods can do to the arteries. The study looked at 24 adults, half with normal cholesterol and half with levels that were moderately high, who were given two high fat meals eaten one week apart. The researchers then added five teaspoons of olive oil for one meal and eight shelled walnuts for the other. The results revealed that both the olive oil and nuts reduced the onset of inflammation following a meal high in saturated fat. But the walnuts also helped preserve the elasticity of the arteries. Almonds have been shown to be just as good at lowering LDL cholesterol as walnuts, and should be just as cardio-protective.

Onions and Garlic

Cook with garlic and onions whenever possible. Both have been shown to cut cholesterol.

Garlic is well known as a cholesterol lowering agent, containing a compound called allicin that changes the way in which the body uses cholesterol, says Stephen Warshafsky MD, assistant professor of medicine at New York Medical College in Valhalla. When Dr Warshafsky analysed data from five of the most reliable scientific studies on garlic and cholesterol, he found that eating one-half to one clove of garlic a day lowered blood cholesterol an average of 9 per cent. Taken fresh or as a supplement it is almost as effective as some cholesterol lowering drugs. Additional benefits are the prevention of clots and positive effects on plaque formation.

Ginger

Although it is much too early to tell if this will benefit those with heart disease, a few preliminary studies suggest that ginger may lower cholesterol and prevent the blood from clotting. Each of these effects may protect the blood vessels from blockage and the damaging effects of blockage such as atherosclerosis, which as we know can lead to a heart attack or stroke.

Oily Fish (salmon, mackerel, herring, sardines, anchovies)

As mentioned previously Eskimos, who eat a reasonably high fat diet, have one of the lowest incidences of heart disease known. This question concerned two investigators, Dr Jorn Dyerberg and H.O. Bang, at the Alberg Hospital in Holland. On examining the incidence of heart disease among Eskimos living in Greenland, they found that when the Eskimos moved to Eastern Canada and ate the same diet as the Canadians, their incidence of heart disease went up to that of their fellow Canadians within one generation. This indicated that their protection against heart disease was not necessarily related to genetics, but must be attributable to some unknown unique factor in their diet. The culprit must have had something to do with the fat content of the diet.

The chemical examination of the oils in the Eskimo diet found that there was a reasonably high concentration of an unusual fatty acid called Omega-3 containing eicosapentaenoic acid, (EPA) and docosahexaenoic acid, (DHA). This fatty acid, which is chemically related to linolenic, linoleic, and arachidonic acids, is apparently manufactured by small unicellular algae that live in the ocean, and has been passed up through the food chain where it is concentrated in the fat tissue of the higher fish.

Cardiovascular Protection

Dr William Connor, professor of medicine and head of the University of Oregon's clinical nutrition section, found that a 10 day diet of salmon, which contains high levels of Omega-3, lowers blood cholesterol by up to 17% per cent in healthy volunteers, and by 20 per cent in patients who have elevated cholesterol. Triglyceride levels in the blood fell by as much as 40 per cent in healthy volunteers and as much as 67 per cent in high triglyceride patients. 'The greatest effect seems to be in patients with elevation of both blood cholesterol and triglyceride levels,' says Dr Connor. 'The higher these levels are when the fish oil program is started, usually the greater the fall.'

In addition, Omega-3 protects against the clumping and unwanted stickiness of a type of blood cell called platelets, which can cause heart attack, stroke, or blockage in other arteries of the body, such as the femoral artery producing a thrombophlebitis. A high concentration of Omega-3 is used by the body to manufacture substances called thromboxane and prostcyclin, which actually prevent platelets from sticking together.

Krill Oil

It has been reported that a daily dose of Krill Oil can be highly beneficial. It is derived from the planktonic crustacean family and it is rich in phospholipids, Omega-3 and antioxidants. It has been observed to lower total bad cholesterol levels by 34 per cent and boost good cholesterol levels by 44 per cent.

Olive Oil

It seems that mono-unsaturated fats reduce the capacity of LDL cholesterol to oxidise, which may explain the protective properties of olive oil. However, extra virgin olive oil also contains around 40 antioxidant phytochemicals, so perhaps these phytochemicals are the factors responsible for the health benefits.

To investigate the effect of antioxidants from olive oil on cholesterol, researchers instructed 16 healthy adults to avoid phenol containing foods such as coffee, tea, wine and vegetables for 4 days. On the fifth day adults consumed 50 ml of virgin olive oil - about 3.3 tablespoons - alone or with bread.

The participants avoided all other foods with phenols for the next 24 hours and then ate their regular diet, supplemented by 25 ml of olive oil daily, for a week. Study volunteers were also told to avoid high fat foods such as butter, margarine, cooking oil, nuts, baked foods and eggs.

Blood samples taken before and during the study revealed higher levels of antioxidant compounds, including vitamin E and phenols, after one week. Similarly, levels of oleic acid, the predominant type of fat in olive oil, as well as of mono-unsaturated fatty acids were higher. These changes were associated with a slower LDL oxidation rate.

In addition to the LDL lowering effect of virgin olive oil, the results suggest that an intake of 25 ml/day could increase the resistance of LDL to oxidation because it becomes richer in oleic acid and antioxidants. These benefits could be achieved by including virgin olive oil daily in our diet.
European Journal of Clinical Nutrition April 2002, 56:114-120

Flax Seed

Flaxseed oil is derived from the seeds of the flax plant. Flaxseed oil and flax seed contain substances that promote good health. Flaxseed oil is rich in alpha-linolenic acid (ALA), an essential fatty acid that appears to be beneficial for a variety of conditions. The body converts ALA to EPA and DHA, the forms more readily used in the body.

Studies suggest that flaxseed oil and other omega-3 fatty acids may be helpful in treating a variety of conditions. The evidence is strongest for heart disease and problems that contribute to heart disease. It is important to maintain an appropriate balance of omega-3 and omega-6 (another essential fatty acid) in the diet as these two substances work together to promote health. These essential fats are both examples of polyunsaturated fatty acids, or PUFAs. Omega-3 fatty acids help reduce inflammation and most omega-6 fatty acids tend to promote inflammation. An inappropriate balance of these essential fatty acids contributes to the development of disease while a proper balance helps maintain and even improve health. A healthy diet should consist of roughly two to four times more omega-6 fatty acids than omega-3 fatty acids. The typical American diet tends to contain 14 to 25 times more omega-6 fatty acids than omega-3 fatty acids and many researchers believe this imbalance is a significant factor in the rising rate of inflammatory disorders in the United States.

Coconut Oil

In the past Coconut Oil has had some bad press due to it getting lumped in with other saturated fats which can cause changes in Cholesterol levels by raising them. It turns out that Coconut Oil raises HDL the 'Good Cholesterol' not LDL 'Bad Cholesterol', now thank goodness we have caught up with the populations around the world who have been eating and applying Coconut Oil for both taste and health reasons for centuries. It's a very healthy fat indeed, which at the very least is a great replacement for spreads and butters.

Coconut Oil has Omega 3 fatty acids as opposed to most cooking oils which contain Omega 6 fatty acids. Omega-3 fatty acids help reduce inflammation and most omega-6 fatty acids tend to promote inflammation. An inappropriate balance of these essential fatty acids contributes to the development of disease while a proper balance helps maintain and even improve health. A healthy diet should consist of roughly two to four times more omega-6 fatty acids than omega-3 fatty acids. The typical western diet tends to contain 14 to 25 times more omega-6 fatty acids than omega-3 fatty acids and many researchers believe this imbalance is a significant factor in the rising rate of inflammatory disorders in the west.

Cooking – Coconut Oil has a higher smoke point which means that it can take higher temperatures than other healthy Omega 3 oils such as Flax and Olive Oil which don't perform well under high heat.

Coconut Oil has antioxidant properties which means that not only is it good for us when consumed or applied, it is stable for over a year at room temperature.

Coconut Oil is unique in being composed of Medium Chain Fatty Acids (MCFA) as opposed to practically all other fats which are Long Chain Fatty Acids (LCFA). It means that Coconut Oil does not turn to fat in the body because it is converted to energy, in fact this happens so quickly that it creates heat in the body to increase metabolism. So ingesting this oil has been shown to help lose body fat, a trial reported by Dr Oz in America points to this with two groups of women on the same diet. One half of the women consumed 2 tablespoons of coconut oil every day for 12 weeks and the other half acted as a control group. It was found that the women who took the coconut oil gained no weight unlike the control group and their abdominal fat was lower. Perhaps some of the weight loss is due to the way Coconut Oil improves a sluggish Thyroid Gland by the production of additional Thyroid hormones. Even in cases of chronic fatigue syndrome and fibromyalgia there are reports of increases in energy.

Soy

Many soya products contain soya protein, which scientists agree helps lower blood cholesterol. Also, many soya products are low in saturated fat and contain soluble fibre, which can also contribute to lowering blood cholesterol. Products providing at least 5g of soya protein per serving will be able to carry this claim on the pack: 'The inclusion of at least 25g of soya protein per day as part of a low saturated fat diet can help reduce blood cholesterol levels.' So says State Registered Dietician and Registered Nutritionist Tanya Carr. Tanya is a member of the British Dietetic

Association and the Nutrition Society, and is a consultant dietician to Alpro (Europe's leading producer of dairy-free products).

Soy reduces cholesterol absorption from the gut, and increases excretion (13-15). The overall effect is a lowering of LDL cholesterol by up to 30 per cent, and a simultaneous increase in HDL cholesterol by up to 15 per cent (16,17-23). The Italian National Health Service now provides soy in the form of textured vegetable protein free to all patients with hypercholesterolaemia (a genetic predisposition to extremely high blood levels of cholesterol). They found that adding soy to a low fat diet dropped cholesterol levels by an impressive 26 per cent (24).

Soy contains Genistein, an isoflavone which has been the subject of well over 300 research papers to date. Its ability to inhibit the growth of certain cell types is cardio-protective. As oxidised cholesterol begins to accumulate in the artery walls, and an atheroma forms, the artery responds by growing more smooth muscle cells in the affected areas. As they grow, they contribute, along with the growing mass of cholesterol, to the gradual blocking of the vessel. Genistein blocks this smooth muscle response (25). It is presumed this plays a role, together with the soy's cholesterol lowering effect and anti-oxidant content, in reducing heart disease in those Far Eastern countries where soy is so widely eaten, and where coronary heart disease is so uncommon.

Despite these assertions, the intake of nonfermented soy should be treated with caution, as this is the fundamental difference between the East and the West. In Asia soy is fermented from six months to three years and is eaten as a condiment, not as a replacement for animal protein as in the West.

Here is an extract on a number of key points concerning the use of Soy by Russell L. Blaylock MD, author of The Taste That Kills and Health and Nutrition Secrets That Can Save Your Life.

'When soybeans are processed, the excitotoxic amino acids (glutamate and aspartate) are not only released, they are concentrated. This is especially so in soy protein isolates and soy protein concentrates, which are used in soy milk.

It has been shown that human blood levels of glutamate increase as much as 20 times on glutamate-loading with concentrations found in such hydrolysed proteins. These high blood levels are transferred into the human brain, especially under certain circumstances. Even in the completely normal brain, glutamate, aspartate and other excitotoxins can enter the brain via the circumventricular organs, which include the hypothalamus. One of the most sensitive structures in the brain is the arcuate nucleus. It is easily destroyed by levels of glutamate found in hydrolysed proteins and this has been proven in laboratory studies.

It is also known that the blood-brain barrier contains glutamate receptors and that free glutamate at these concentrations can open the barrier, allowing these high levels of glutamate freely to enter the brain.

It is also known that a multitude of conditions open the barrier, including strokes (both gross and silent), brain injury, brain tumours, certain pesticides, mercury, lead, autoimmune disorders (lupus, rheumatoid arthritis, etc), radio frequency radiation (cell phones), seizures, multiple sclerosis and infections. Anyone with these or related conditions should avoid products that contain high levels of excitotoxins, such as hydrolysed soy products. This constitutes a large percentage of the population.

Experiments have also shown that early exposure to glutamate can alter – permanently -the baby's vascular reactivity. This would have major implications in cardiovascular disease. Likewise, early exposure to higher levels of glutamate, equal to that of food-based excitotoxins, results in behavioural problems, endocrine disruption, increased susceptibility to seizures early in life and alterations in lipid profiles that increase the likelihood of cardiovascular disease later in life. In fact, newer studies have shown that elevated blood glutamate significantly increases free radical generation in the endothelial lining of blood vessels - the very mechanism that causes atherosclerosis.

Recent research has also shown that many tissues and organs in the body contain glutamate receptors and that overstimulation of these receptors can cause a number of clinical problems. For example, glutamate receptor stimulation of pulmonary tissues can result in bronchiospasm (as in asthma) and worsening of pulmonary function in cases of lung diseases. The heart muscle and heart conduction system (AV and SA nodes) also contain numerous glutamate receptors. The pancreas (islets of Langerhans) also contains abundant glutamate receptors, and explains the resulting diabetes.

Even more frightening is the recent discovery that glutamate greatly enhances the growth of a number of cancers, especially brain cancers such as glioblastoma and the malignant astrocytoma. Breast, lung and ovarian cancers have also been shown to spread and metastasise faster when glutamate levels are elevated. This has been proven and is beyond dispute.'

Blaylock adds that we know that glutamate toxicity is greatly increased under certain conditions, which include low magnesium levels, deficient mitochondrial energy production such as occurs in hypoglycaemia, and mitochondrial disease during ageing, together with all of the neurodegenerative diseases i.e. most chronic diseases plus Alzheimer's, Parkinson's and amyotrophic lateral sclerosis (ALS), the latter known also as 'Lou Gehrig's disease' – a progressive neurodegenerative disease that affects nerve cells in the brain and the spinal cord. An increase in glutamate toxicity also occurs during inflammation and when associated with other toxins including mercury, lead, cadmium, aluminium, pesticides, fluoride and industrial chemicals. This would affect tens of millions of Americans, who should be avoiding soy products.

'Soybeans,' Blaylock continues, 'and especially their hydrolysed and processed products, contain high levels of manganese, aluminium and fluoride, all of which are powerful cell toxins, especially for brain cells.

Recent studies have shown that when aluminium is combined with fluoride, which occurs very easily, brain levels of aluminium are doubled. Extensive research connects aluminium in the brain with most of the neurodegenerative diseases. When hydrolysed as in soy milk, the fluoride and aluminium easily bind, forming neurotoxic fluoroaluminum compounds. The concentration at which this occurs is 0.5 ppm, a very small concentration. Fluoroaluminum compounds interact with G-proteins, which are common cell communication systems especially in the brain and operate most of the glutamanergic receptors in the brain (glutamate receptors).

I would call attention to a most important study reported in the Journal of the American College of Nutrition in the year 2000. It describes a 25-year study of middle-aged individuals consuming a diet containing tofu, which found a strong association with brain atrophy and cognitive impairment and the consumption of this soy product. Brain atrophy was determined by MRI scans. In fact, low brain weight was seen in 12 per cent of men consuming the lowest amount of tofu and 40 percent consuming the highest amount. This indicates a dose-response effect, making a stronger case of neurotoxicity'.

It seems that we must be careful to take into account that soy based products which have been demonstrated to work against high cholesterol may do so at a price, with growing evidence, quite apart from the GM debate, that there are a number of potentially serious side effects.

Minerals for the heart

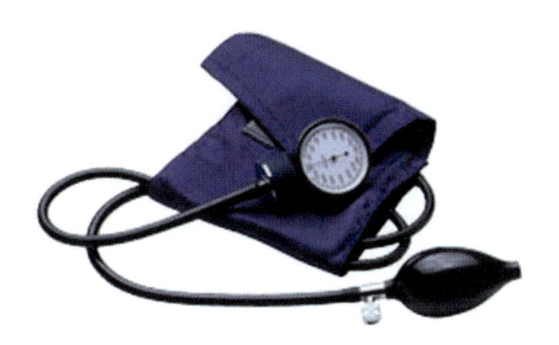

Sodium and potassium

The modern diet, which contains too much sodium and too little potassium, contributes to the age-related rise in blood pressure so common in the West. It is a major contributory factor to heart attacks and strokes, particularly in the overweight.

Top Potassium Foods

Potassium rich foods include:-					
Lentils	730mg	1 cup	Banana	450mg	medium
Kidney beans	700mg	1 cup	Avocado	550mg	half
Prune juice	700mg	8oz	Carrot (raw)	232mg	medium
Tomato juice	652mg	6oz	Milk	381mg	8oz
Chick peas	470mg	1 cup	Orange juice	474mg	8oz

Magnesium

This essential mineral protects the arterial linings from stress caused by sudden blood pressure changes, which are at the root of many cardiovascular disorders.

Magnesium salts are a major component in hard water, and people who live in areas where the drinking water is hard have a reduced risk of heart disease. Magnesium depletion causes atheroma and magnesium supplements clean the arteries out again. This is thought to be because depletion leads to an increased free radical synthesis and increased oxidation in the tissues. Magnesium deficiency may be a major cause of fatal cardiac arrhythmia, hypertension, and sudden cardiac arrest.

Sources

Magnesium is found in most foods especially dairy products, fish, meat, and seafood. Other rich food sources include apples, apricots, avocados, bananas, blackstrap molasses, brewer's yeast, brown rice, cantaloupe, dulse, figs, garlic, grapefruit, green leafy vegetables, kelp, lemons, lima beans, millet, nuts, peaches, black-eyed peas, salmon, sesame seeds, soybeans, tofu, watercress, wheat and whole grains.

Calcium

Calcium deficiency can lead to elevated blood cholesterol, heart palpitations and hypertension.

Sources

Calcium is found in milk and dairy foods, salmon (with bones), sardines, seafood, and green leafy vegetables. Food sources include almonds, asparagus, blackstrap molasses, brewer's yeast, broccoli, buttermilk, cabbage, carob, cheese, dulse, figs, goat's milk, kale, kelp, oats, prunes, sesame seeds, soybeans, tofu, and watercress.

Copper

Copper depletion is quite common, and has been linked to an increased risk of heart disease. The level of copper in the body is related to the levels of zinc and vitamin C. Copper levels are reduced if large amounts of zinc and vitamin C are consumed. If copper intake is too high, levels of vitamin C and zinc drop.

The consumption of high amounts of fructose can significantly worsen a copper deficiency. In a study by the US Department of Agriculture, people who obtained 20 per cent of their daily calories from fructose showed decreased levels of red blood cell superoxide dismutase (SOD), a copper-dependent enzyme critical to antioxidant protection within the red blood cells.

Sources

Food sources include almonds, avocados, barley, beans, beets, blackstrap molasses, broccoli, garlic, lentils, liver, mushrooms, nuts, oats, oranges, pecans, radishes, raisins, salmon, seafood, soybeans, and green leafy vegetables.

Selenium

As mentioned in the section on antioxidants, selenium's function is to inhibit the oxidation of lipids. It is a vital antioxidant, especially when combined with vitamin E.

Selenium deficiency has been linked to high cholesterol and heart disease. Veterinarians are familiar with heart problems caused by selenium depletion in cattle and livestock. Humans are equally susceptible – although it is only in areas with an extremely low intake of selenium, such as Keshan in China, where cause and effect are relatively easy to single out. In the UK, the Scots are particularly likely to be low in this essential trace mineral.

Taking selenium supplements can lead to reductions in total blood cholesterol and improvements in HDL levels. Recent research by Margaret

Rayman from the University of Surrey recruited 501 subjects aged between 60 and 74. the subjects were divided into four groups, which received 100, 200, or 300 mcg of high-selenium yeast supplements, or placebos for six months. People taking 100mcg of selenium had an average 8.5mg/dl decrease in their cholesterol levels, and those taking 200mcg of selenium had an average 9.7mg/dl decrease in their cholesterol. Those taking 300mcg of selenium daily had just a 2.7mg/dl decrease in their cholesterol. Interestingly this group was the only one to have a significant increase in HDL cholesterol – an average of 2.3mg.dl.

> Reference: Rayman MP, Stranges S Griffin BA, et al. Effect of supplementation with high-slenium yeast on plasma lipids. Annals of Internal Medicine, 2011;154:656-665

Sources

Food sources include brazil nuts, brewer's yeast, broccoli, brown rice, chicken, dairy products, dulse, garlic, kelp, liver, molasses, onions, salmon, seafood, tuna, vegetables, wheat germ, and whole grains.

Silicon

Silicon has been seen to inhibit atheromas (fatty deposits or plaques resulting from atherosclerosis) in rabbits fed an atheromatous diet, making plaque formation rare and lipid deposits more superficial. Silicon is essential for the integrity of the tunica intima, the inner lining of arterial tissue. Cardiovascular health requires silicon for the generation of elastin, the tissue comprising the inner lining of arteries and capillaries. Diseased arteries are severely deficient in silicon.

Dietary fibre has been found to help prevent atherosclerosis by reducing cholesterol, blood lipids and binding bile acids.

Sources

Whole grain cereals (especially oats) and their products (especially beer), rice, Kenyan beans, French beans, runner beans, spinach, dried fruit, bananas and red lentils, plus mineral water.

Germanium

This mineral improves cellular oxygenation. A Japanese scientist, Kazuhiko Asai, found that an intake of 100 to 300 milligrams of germanium per day improved many illnesses, including elevated cholesterol.

Sources

Food sources include garlic, shiitake mushrooms, onions and the herbs aloe vera, comfrey, ginseng, and suma.

A mineral to beware of-

Iron

A vital mineral in the production of haemoglobin and myoglobin (the form of haemoglobin found in muscle tissue) and the oxygenation of red blood cells.

However, because iron is stored in the body, excessive iron intake can also cause problems. Too much iron in the tissues and organs leads to the production of free radicals and increases the need for vitamin E.

Unless iron deficiency is diagnosed as anaemia, supplementation should be used judiciously. Special attention should be given to men and post-menopausal women: there is some evidence that in men with very high iron levels in the blood, the risk of heart disease can be increased by as much as 100 per cent. Men should probably only take iron supplements if there is a clear evidence of iron deficiency anaemia.*

Sources

Iron is found in eggs, fish, liver, meat, poultry, green leafy vegetables, whole grains and enriched breads and cereals. Other food sources include almonds, avocados, beets, blackstrap molasses, brewer's yeast, dates, dulse, kelp, kidney and lima beans, lentils, millet, peaches, pears, dried prunes, pumpkins, raisins, rice and wheat bran, sesame seeds, soybeans, and watercress.

*As a postscript on iron, beware of aluminium which displaces iron from its carrier molecules. Increased free iron could contribute to increased tissue damage in vessel walls. Chronic aluminium exposure from sources such as antiperspirants, antacids, antiseptics and soda cans is likely to be cardio-toxic.

Amino Acids and the heart

Carnitine

Its main function in the body is to help transport long chain fatty acids, which are burned within the cells to provide energy. This is a major source of energy for the muscles. Carnitine thus increases the use of fat as an energy source. This prevents fatty build-up, especially in the heart, liver, and skeletal muscles. Carnitine reduces the health risks posed by poor fat metabolism associated with diabetes, inhibits alcohol-induced fattyliver, and lessens the risk of heart disorders. Studies have shown that patients who take supplemental carnitine in the form of L-carnitine soon after suffering a heart attack may be less likely to suffer a subsequent heart attack, die of heart disease, or experience chest pain and abnormal heart rhythms. In addition, people with coronary artery disease who use L-carnitine along with standard medication may be able to sustain physical activity for longer periods of time.

Carnitine has the ability to lower blood triglyceride levels, aid in weight loss, and enhance the effectiveness of the antioxidant vitamins E and C.

Sources

Carnitine can be manufactured by the body if sufficient amounts of iron, vitamin B1 (thiamine), vitamin B6 (pyridoxine), and the amino acids lysine and methionine are available. The synthesis of carnitine also depends on the presence of adequate levels of vitamin C.

Food sources are primarily meats and other foods of animal origin.

Many cases of carnitine deficiency have been identified as partly genetic in origin, resulting from an inherited defect in carnitine synthesis. Possible symptoms of deficiency include confusion, heart pain, muscle weakness, and obesity. Because of their generally greater muscle mass, men need more carnitine than women do. Vegetarians are more likely than nonvegetarians to be deficient in carnitine because it is not found in vegetable protein. Moreover, neither methionine nor lysine, two of the key constituents from which the body makes carnitine, are obtainable from vegetable sources in sufficient amounts.

For vegetarians in particular, L-carnitine supplementation should be considered (300mg three times a day).

Lysine and Proline

The amino acids lysine and proline were favourites of the late Nobel Prize winner Dr Linus Pauling. They are thought to act as a kind of arterial Teflon, stopping apolipoprotein B sticking to the artery wall. Used with high doses of vitamin C and other antioxidants, they have reportedly achieved cures in patients with advanced coronary artery disease, relieving the symptoms of angina within a few months.

Lysine helps in collagen formation, tissue repair, and lowers high serum triglyceride levels. Lysine is an essential amino acid which means it cannot be manufactured in the body. It is therefore vital that adequate amounts be included in the diet.

Sources

Food sources of lysine include cheese, eggs, fish, lima beans, milk, potatoes, red meat, soy products, and yeast.

Proline helps in the strengthening of the heart muscle, and works with vitamin C to promote healthy connective tissue. Proline improves skin texture by aiding in the production of collagen and reducing the loss of collagen through the ageing process.

Sources

Proline is obtained primarily from meat sources.

Chitosan, a polymer of glucosamine, demonstrates cholesterol lowering action within the liver, capable of reversing adverse changes provoked by high cholesterol diets. Total levels of LDL cholesterol and triglycerides have been shown to be lowered with the use of chitosan, whilst elevating high-density lipids (HDL). Chitosan is a compound for lowering fat intake into your system as it attracts and absorbs fat molecules from the food source passing them harmlessly through the body.

Caution

Firstly, you should <u>not</u> take chitosan with any fat-soluble vitamins such as E or A, nor with Evening Primrose Oil, Omega-3 Fish Oil, nor Cod Liver Oil. The reason is obvious: chitosan will not differentiate 'good' from 'bad' fats and will roll them up and out of the body. The second point is that chitosan does not remove fat already deposited in the body, so sensible eating, coupled with exercise, is crucial to success.

Arginine, increases nitric oxide levels, a blood vessel dilator and clot buster produced in endothelial cells by the enzyme nitric oxide synthase. In their book, 'The Arginine Solution' Drs Robert Fried and Woodson C. Merrell note that as people age and develop disorders such as hypertension, hypercholesterolemia, and artherosclerosis their ability to make sufficient amounts of nitric oxide from arginine is impaired, contributing to a decline in their cardiovascular health.

Sources

Most protein foods and carob, chocolate, nuts, seeds, beans, oats, peanuts, and wheat and wheat germ.

Creatine is naturally produced in the human body from amino acids primarily in the kidney and liver. It is transported in the blood for use by muscles. Approximately 95% of the human body's total creatine is located in skeletal muscle.

Creatine is not an essential nutrient, as it is manufactured in the human body from L-Arginine, glycine and L-Methionine. If you are taking statin drugs and experiencing any of the classic side effects such as myalgia, weakness and lethargy then Creatine supplementation should be considered. It is thought that one of the effects of statin drugs may be a decrease in intracellular creatine in muscle, similar to the toxic effects of glucocorticoids and clyclosporine.

A recent study performed at the John Hopkins School of Public Health (Ann Intern Med. 2010 Nov 16;153(10);690-2) found creatine highly effective for reducing the side effects of statin drugs. Although the study sample was small at just 12 patients identified as intolerant of several different statin drugs, amazingly the study found that Creatine loading followed by maintenance Creatine therapy totally prevented myopathy symptoms in eight out of 10 patients receiving statins. More telling of the profound effect of the Creatine: all patients went on to develop myopathy symptoms while receiving statins alone; which went away after Creatine was reintroduced. This is highly significant and should have the same weighting on treating and prevention of statin side effects as supplementation with CoQ10. One last point is that vegetarians may be at higher risk of creatine depletion because in addition to biosynthesise from essential amino acids the primary food source of creatine is meat.

Caution Creatine supplementation cannot be recommended during pregnancy or breastfeeding due to a lack of scientific information.

Vitamins Vital for the heart

We have already covered vitamins A, C and E in the section on antioxidants, and folic acid, vitamin B6 and vitamin B12 under methyl donors, so the next heart friendly vitamins include the following:

Vitamin D

Low levels of vitamin D may increase the risk of calcium build-up in the arteries, a significant component of atherosclerotic plaque. This fat-soluble vitamin is also involved in the regulation of the heartbeat.

Sources

Food sources include fish liver oils, fatty saltwater fish, dairy products, and eggs. It is found in butter, cod liver oil, liver, milk, oatmeal, salmon, sardines, sweet potatoes, tuna, and vegetable oils.

Vitamin D is also formed in the body in response to the action of sunlight on the skin.*

> * Some cholesterol-lowering drugs interfere with the absorption of vitamin D.

Vitamin B1 (Thiamine)

Among patients hospitalised with heart failure, about one in three has deficient levels of thiamine, although thiamine deficiency was less common among those patients who were taking vitamin supplements, according to a new Canadian study. Researchers measured the thiamine levels of 100 consecutively admitted patients with heart failure. They also measured the thiamine levels of 50 healthy people. The heart failure patients were almost three times as likely to deficient in thiamine as the control subjects. (26) 16/12/2004 – 'High doses of vitamin B1, or thiamine, could lower cholesterol in diabetes patients and help prevent heart disease,' say UK researchers. The findings, based on a rat model of diabetes, may be important in the face of the rising incidence of diabetes around the globe.

Diabetes increases the risk of heart disease two to three fold in men and three to five fold in women. The increased risk is linked to high levels of cholesterol and lipids in the blood.

In another study, researchers at the University of Essex are confident that high doses of thiamine could also help to reverse the increases in blood cholesterol and lipid levels.

They studied control and diabetic rats for 24 weeks with and without oral high-dose therapy with thiamine.

'We found that thiamine therapy (70 mg/kg) prevented diabetes-induced increases in plasma cholesterol and triglycerides in diabetic rats but did not reverse the diabetes-induced decrease of HDL,' they report in Diabetologia (DOI: 10.1007/s00125-004-1582-5). Thiamine also normalised the food intake of diabetic rats.

Lead researcher Professor Paul Thornalley commented, ' There will of course be clinical trials to investigate further the findings we have made using an experimental model of diabetes. However, given the continuing toll of heart disease in diabetic patients, and the emerging benefits of thiamine therapy for diabetics suffering from kidney disease - as reported by our research group last year - I would strongly suggest that those with diabetes are given thiamine supplements.'

Sources

The richest food sources of thiamine include brown rice, egg yolks, fish, legumes, liver, peanuts, peas, pork, poultry, rice bran, wheat germ, and whole grains. Other sources are asparagus, brewer's yeast, broccoli, Brussels sprouts, dulse, kelp, most nuts, oatmeal, plums, dried prunes, raisins, spirulina, and watercress.

Vitamin B3 (Niacin)

Niacin is a natural cholesterol lowering agent that, alone, has been shown to outperform prescriptive drugs in mild and even moderate cases. It helps your body to work on the cellular level and increases the health of the digestive system, improves circulation, promotes healthy skin and the sound functioning of your nervous system.

Niacin supplements are available as nicotinamide or nicotinic acid. Nicotinamide is the form of niacin typically used in nutritional supplements and in food fortification. Nicotinic acid is available over the counter and with a prescription as a cholesterol lowering agent.

According to Jane Higdon PhD of the Linus Pauling Institute at Oregon State University,

'Pharmacological doses of nicotinic acid, but not nicotinamide, have been known to reduce serum cholesterol since 1955. Only one randomized placebo-controlled multicenter trial examined the effect of nicotinic acid therapy alone (3 grams daily) on outcomes of cardiovascular disease. The Coronary Drug Project (CDP) followed over 8,000 men with a previous myocardial infarction (heart attack) for 6 years. In the group that took 3 grams of nicotinic acid daily, total blood cholesterol decreased by an average of 10%, triglycerides decreased by 26%, recurrent nonfatal myocardial infarction decreased by 27%, and cerebrovascular events (stroke + transient ischemic attacks) decreased by 26% compared to the placebo group.'

Sources

Niacin and niacinamide are found in beef liver, brewer's yeast, broccoli, carrots, cheese, corn flour, dates, eggs, fish, milk, peanuts, pork, potatoes, tomatoes, wheat germ, and whole wheat products.

Cautions

People who are pregnant or who suffer from diabetes, glaucoma, gout, liver disease, or peptic ulcers should use niacin supplements with caution. Amounts over 500 milligrams daily may cause liver damage if taken for prolonged periods.

Quick note on supplements versus prescription drugs. The majority of natural ingredients you see I have listed have more than one mode of action on more than one of the major mechanisms of imbalance within the body. When you see natural formulas which appear in the market place you will undoubtedly find there is an overlapping of mechanisms of action which tend to have a synergistic effect on the causes of potentially dangerous lipid profiles, and in some cases they can have dramatic results. Such characteristics are typically lacking in prescription drugs, which generally target only one mechanism, and when they interact it is often in a negative, rather than a synergistic fashion. Most drug trials are conducted with either healthy generally young individuals or an effected group with what ever the drug mechanism is targeted at. Apart from known contraindications and adverse reactions of all drugs, the fact that a huge number of the population are on an age related polypharmacy, (administration of many drugs together) which are unique to the individual, makes natural supplements versus drugs an even more important distinction.

Foods to avoid X

Sugar

Put simply, refined sugar overstimulates the hormone insulin, which in turn stimulates HMG-CoA reductase (an enzyme responsible for cholesterol synthesis inside each cell). As insulin speeds up the enzyme activity within the cholesterol manufacturing pipeline, it leads to a build up and surplus within each cell. At this point there is no need for the cell to retrieve any from the bloodstream and cholesterol begins to build up in the blood. Reduce insulin and immediately the signal that causes an increase in cholesterol synthesis is silenced and the cells begin to harvest the necessary cholesterol directly from the blood, causing blood levels to drop. Excess insulin also inhibits the release of glucagon. Glucagon's job is to restore blood sugar levels for optimal brain function. Glucagon inhibits the activity of HMG-CoA reductase. So by increasing the hormone glucagon you decrease the cholesterol producing machinery inside the cells, forcing LDL receptors to rush to the cell surface in an effort to pull cholesterol from the blood and restore the appropriate balance.

Bad fats

As previously mentioned, saturated fat, the kind found primarily in red meats, butter and other animal foods, is incredibly bad for the heart. Study after study has shown the more saturated fat people get in their diets, the higher their risk of heart disease.

Foods high in saturated fat raise levels of artery-clogging low density lipoprotein (LDL) cholesterol, says Michael Gaziano MD, director of cardiovascular epidemiology at Brigham and Women's Hospital in Boston. What's more, foods high in saturated fat are often rich in cholesterol as well. The danger is so great that the American Heart Association recommends that we get no more (and preferably less) than 10 per cent of our calories from saturated fat. It means that if a person's daily calorie intake is 2,000 calories, the daily limit for saturated fat is 22 grams. In essence it means that in addition to having fruits, vegetables, and other low-fat foods, you could have as an example 3 ounces of extra-lean ground beef (5 grams of saturated fat), a serving of macaroni cheese (6 grams), and six onion rings (10 grams).

But even this modest amount of saturated fat is not ideal. 'Your best bet for lowering heart disease risk is to reduce the amount of saturated fat in your diet to less than 10 per cent of your total calories,' says Dr Gaziano.

Another type of problem fat, called trans-fatty acids, which are found mainly in margarine, were meant to be a healthy alternative to saturated fat in butter. Studies have shown, however, that it may not be the best choice.

In fact, trans-fatty acids may be just as bad as the saturated fat in butter, says Christopher Gardner PhD, research fellow at the Stanford University Center for Research in Disease Prevention in Palo Alto, California. So you don't want to eat a lot of them. And it's not only margarine that may be a problem. Many biscuits, cakes, and other snack foods contain partially hydrogenated oil, which is also high in trans-fatty acids.

Natural v Synthetic

This example serves to highlight how far the food industry, with its routine manipulation of chemicals, has taken us away from whole foods and natural products.

Which would you rather eat a little of? ***Reduce or avoid all processed foods.***

Butter:	Margarine:
milk fat (cream), a little salt	Edible oils, edible fats, salt or potassium chloride, ascorbyl palmitate, butylated hydroxyanisole, phospholipids, tert-butylhydroquinone, mono- and di-glycerides of fat-forming fatty acids, disodium guanylate, diacetyltartaric and fatty acid esters of glycerol, Propyl, octyl or dodecyl gallate (or mixtures thereof), tocopherols, propylene glycol mono- and di-esters, sucrose esters of fatty acids, curcumin, annatto extracts, tartaric acid, 3,5,trimethylhexanal, ß-apo-carotenoic acid methyl or ethyl ester, skim milk powder, xanthophylls, canthaxanthin, vitamins A and D.

Coffee?

Coffee is a stimulant that affects the adrenals, which in consequence use up more vital vitamin C.

However, a report in the American Journal of Clinical Nutrition seems to contradict numerous studies that have suggested that coffee is bad for you and shows that longer term, drinking coffee cuts the risk of death from CVD. Based on a study of over 41,000 women followed for 15 years, it found risk of death from cardiovascular disease (CVD) was 24% lower among those consuming 1 to 3 cups of coffee daily, which was confirmed by other studies on men and women. Preventing cardiovascular disease at the cellular level, just one cup of coffee inhibited platelet aggregation within one hour, regardless of its caffeine content. The analysis, part of the Iowa Women's Health Study, found that up to 60 per cent of antioxidants in the diet may come from coffee.

It is a common misconception that coffee raises blood pressure and increases the risk of CVD. In fact scientific studies show that coffee's compounds lower blood pressure over the long term, decrease the risk of cardiovascular disease, and may reduce the risk of stroke. It is true that drinking coffee can raise the blood pressure briefly, right after consumption. But its compounds have a longer term benefit: daily coffee consumption decreases blood pressure readings after just 8 weeks, which is believed to be a result of the beneficial action of chlorogenic acids on the arteries.

Active parts of coffee include caffeine and polyphenols. Polyphenols are also found in red wine which, as previously discussed, has been linked to a reduction in the risk of cardiovascular disease. Further studies found that regular coffee consumption improved inflammation and HDL cholesterol, and decreased coronary calcification.

My view at this stage is that if you already drink coffee, then moderate consumption may be beneficial provided adequate amounts of vitamin C are consumed. If you do not drink coffee you do not need to start in order to gain antioxidant protection. Just take a look at the antioxidant section for better alternatives.

Exercise

What's the best type of exercise for my heart?
Aerobic exercise causes you to breathe more deeply and makes your heart work harder to pump blood. Aerobic exercise also raises your heart rate (which also burns calories). Examples of aerobic exercise include walking, jogging, running, swimming and bicycling Most studies have been performed on aerobic exercises, such as jogging, running and aerobics. Aerobic exercises appear to benefit cholesterol the most, by lowering LDL by 5 to 10% and raising HDL cholesterol by 3 to 6%.

How much exercise do I need?
In general, if you haven't been exercising, try to work up to 30 minutes, 4 to 6 times a week. Your doctor may make a different recommendation based on your health. If you can't carry on a conversation while you exercise, you may be overdoing it. It is best to alternate exercise days with rest days to prevent injuries.

Stress reduction

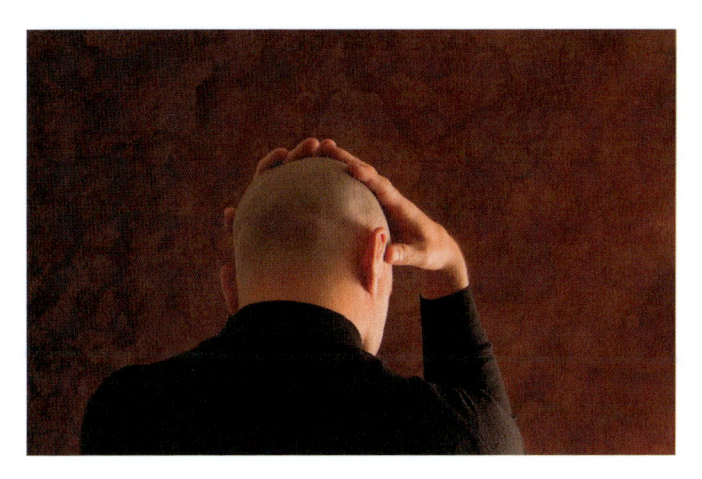

Anyone who says they are not stressed is not strictly telling the truth: we have stress hormones circulating in our bloodstream in different amounts as long as we have a pulse!

The fact is that our hormones have not evolved from caveman times when 'Fight or Flight' meant a choice - are we going to run from the Sabre Toothed Tiger or fight it?

Today, however, if we are stuck in a traffic jam and about to miss that urgent appointment, our stress hormones are rushing around and it's a bit like slipping our body's clutch with our foot on the accelerator. Our adrenals pump out cortisol which galvanises the body during stress. The heart speeds up, blood pressure rises and our demand for energy means we switch from eating proteins towards sugars to fuel the muscles. Under normal circumstances, after the stressful event has passed, another hormone called DHEA acts like a handbrake to reduce the cortisol levels and the adrenals go into a resting phase.

So what happens if the stress is ongoing? Firstly, the physiological effects of sustained stress can cause cravings for sugar which wildly affects our blood sugar levels and takes us on a roller coaster ride. We may find ourselves waking at 3 am, just as if a boiler timer had gone off, because of the adrenals shifting out of their 24-hour rhythm and starting the anabolic cycle too soon. We don't reach the restorative REM (rapid eye movement) state even when we are asleep, so we feel TATT (tired all the time). Our immune function becomes impaired and, in addition to potential depression, we are liable to get allergies of all kinds and osteoporosis. Wow! we should have a national flag day for the adrenals to draw attention to the physiological effects of stress.

Worthwhile Strategies.

Look up 'Glycaemic index of foods' as a search on the internet. You will find lists of foods with a Glycaemic rating: the higher the number, the faster the carbohydrate breaks down to sugar – and the greater the stress.

Eating protein instead of or with carbohydrates will reduce the blood sugar load on the body.

Before retiring to bed eat a couple of oat cakes, which will help to maintain blood sugar levels whilst asleep and prevent your body waking you with a 'starvation warning'.

The adrenals use more vitamin C than any other organ for their size, so if you find you are bruising easily or have bleeding gums it could be a good idea to supplement with this vital vitamin.

B vitamins are also important, in particular B5 pantothenic acid. Please note that all the B vitamins and vitamin C are water soluble, which means your body cannot store them, so it is always better to take smaller doses spread out through the day.

Ginseng also helps the adrenals as it is known as an adaptogen, which means that it can help to reset the timing of when the adrenals should be working.

If your mind will not switch off when you should be sleeping, try a Bach flower remedy called White Chestnut taken as four drops before bedtime.

Do not take stimulants such as caffeine in coffee.

Never watch the news before retiring to bed - light hearted TV, and soft music only!

Gentle regular exercise is good for stress; exercise which is too vigorous is not.

Seek out some of the complementary therapies such as Aromatherapy, Acupuncture, Reiki, etc.

Meditation groups are worthwhile, for example Yoga or Tai Chi.

Always remember to schedule some 'Me Time'.

Connect with Nature and learn to become aware of your breathing.

If something causes you stress and you cannot change it, then change your attitude towards it.

Finally………Thought for the Day – By Brahma Kumaris:

'Instead of becoming disheartened by any type of upheaval, become one with a big heart'.

Traditional Chinese Medicine (TCM) and the heart

In TCM it is said the 'heart houses the mind'. The heart is considered the main organ governing mental activities and its links to the brain. Put another way, there is a mutual effect and correlation between the heart dominating the vessels and the vessels supplying the mind.

To give an example of how emotional stress can have a physiological effect, here is an extract from an article published in the Daily Mail in March 2006 entitled ' Row with your loved one hurts the heart' where it was reported that a three year study of older married couples found their arteries hardened and narrowed after they were involved in arguments, raising their risk of heart disease.

For women, this happened when the row took on a hostile nature. But for men it occurred only when either they or their wife acted in a dominating and controlling manner. American scientists asked 150 couples in their

60s and 70s to discuss a sore topic such as money or their in-laws for six minutes. Each conversation was observed by psychologists who gave a point score for friendly, hostile or dominant behaviour. Two days later the couples were given CAT scans to show the extent of atherosclerosis. The results revealed that the couples who had the most stormy rows showed the most signs of having narrowed arteries.

Tim Smith, Professor of Psychology at the University of Utah, said, 'Disagreements are an unavoidable fact of relationships, but the way we talk during disagreements gives us an opportunity to do something healthy. If you were concerned about men's heart health, you would ask couples to find ways to talk about disagreements without trying to control each other. If you were concerned about women's heart health, you would encourage couples to find ways to have disagreements that were not hostile.'

Dr Stephen Gascoigne, a medically qualified acupuncturist and author, states that the best way of reducing cholesterol levels is to 'deal with reactions to stress and to strengthen the function of the liver and digestion.' You are as unique as your fingerprint, so an holistic approach to treating the underlying imbalances specific to the individual is likely to be more successful than treating the symptoms.

In terms of TCM, raised cholesterol levels usually correspond to phlegm in the blood, says Dr Gascoigne. 'It is important to consider particularly the function of the spleen and the blood and its related organs – heart and kidney.' This may sound like strange terminology to anyone not familiar with Chinese medicine, and I do not propose to go into more detail in this book, but suffice to say that a TCM practitioner will assess the balance of energy in three ways: asking about the symptoms, feeling the pulse, and looking at the tongue. Further information is obtained by observing the face and complexion, or sometimes by physical examination. A diagnosis can then be made and treatment applied using acupuncture and herbs.

Iridology

I have included iridology in this section even though it offers a diagnostic protocol only, owing to its often miraculous ability to pinpoint health issues throughout the body.

An ancient Chinese text says, 'The liver opens into the eyes', and it is as though the heart of each person speaks through the eyes. Iridology is the study of the coloured part of the eye (called the iris) to determine potential health problems. Iridologists believe that changing patterns and markings in the iris can be used to reveal emerging conditions in every part of the body and to identify inherited weaknesses that may lead to physical and emotional disorders. In this example we see a person who may be exhibiting high cholesterol levels with an observation by an iridologist of something called the sodium/cholesterol ring.

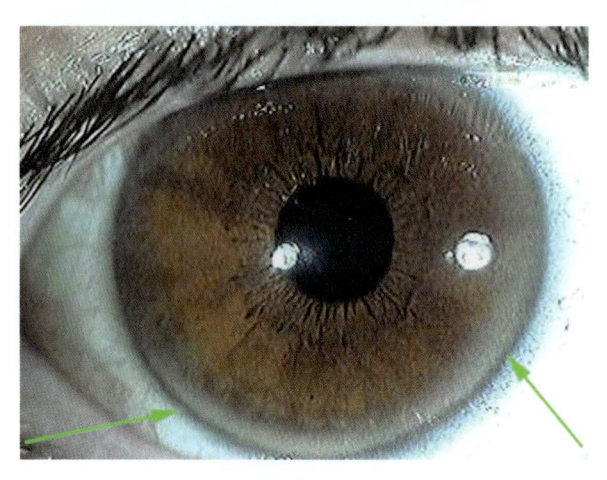

SODIUM / CHOLESTEROL RING

According to an iridologist this picture is a sign of a chemical imbalance in the body, pertaining to non organic sodium excess, calcium out of solution, and high cholesterol and high triglycerides in the blood. Cholesterol Ring is also a non-specific liver marking. It may transpire when hepatopathies (liver disease), diabetes mellitus or hypo-activity of the thyroid are present.

When there is a problem with inorganic sodium and excessive fats in the body, there may be hardening of the arteries, calcium spurs and deposits, joint problems and so on. This does not necessarily mean that the blood levels of cholesterol are high but indicates there is an imbalance of fat metabolism. The cholesterol ring is a white, opaque ring that appears around the outer edge of the iris either partially or wholly.

Homoeopathy

Although few studies have examined the effectiveness of specific homoeopathic remedies, professional homoeopaths would recommend appropriate treatments to reduce the risk of atherosclerosis based on their knowledge and experience. Homoeopathic prescriptions for atherosclerosis would include remedies to lower high blood pressure and cholesterol. In homoeopathic terms, a person's constitutional type is his or her physical, emotional, and intellectual makeup. An experienced homoeopath would assess all of these factors when determining the most appropriate remedy for the individual.

Massage and Physical Therapy

Massage has a relaxing effect and has been shown to reduce stress-related hormone levels. Lowering stress hormone levels positively influences cholesterol and blood pressure and may therefore reduce the risk of heart disease. In addition, relaxation techniques may help individuals comply with habits necessary to reduce the risk of atherosclerosis, such as dieting, quitting smoking, and exercising.

Chapter 5

HOW *YOU* CAN BEAT HIGH CHOLESTEROL

Following on from the detail of what to pay attention to in the last chapter, as promised we arrive at concise information for you to maintain a healthy heart naturally.

Let's look at the risk factors for Cardiovascular Disease (CVD) once more:
- Smoking - increases arterial oxidation.
- Dyslipidaemia – high cholesterol levels with high LDL and low HDL, high triglycerides – lipid profile may respond to increased intake of plant sterols, probiotics, vitamin B3, fibre and fish oils + further natural ways listed throughout chapter 4.
- Diabetes/Insulin Resistance – dysglycaemia can lead to dyslipidaemia and increased inflammation.
- Hypertension – reduced by increased fruit and vegetable consumption, garlic, CoQ10 and fish oil supplementation + stress management.
- Obesity – those with high waist circumference i.e. 'apple shaped' more at risk of CVD.
- High homocysteine levels – modulated by B6, B12, folate, magnesium and trimethylglycine (TMG).
- High ferritin – iron should not be supplemented unless deficient.
- High fibrinogen – can encourage blood clot formation – can be moderated by B6, bromelain (a digestive enzyme from pineapple that assists in the breakdown of food proteins into amino acids and polypeptides), and garlic.
- High C-Reactive Protein – indicative of inflammation and possible arterial damage. Has been associated with low B6 levels. Explore Serrapeptase.

- Oxidative stress – vitamin E complex with tocotrienols, CoQ10, lycopene, and Oligomeric Proanthocyanidins (OPCs) give antioxidant protection (see full list of antioxidants in chapter 4).

The Mediterranean Diet

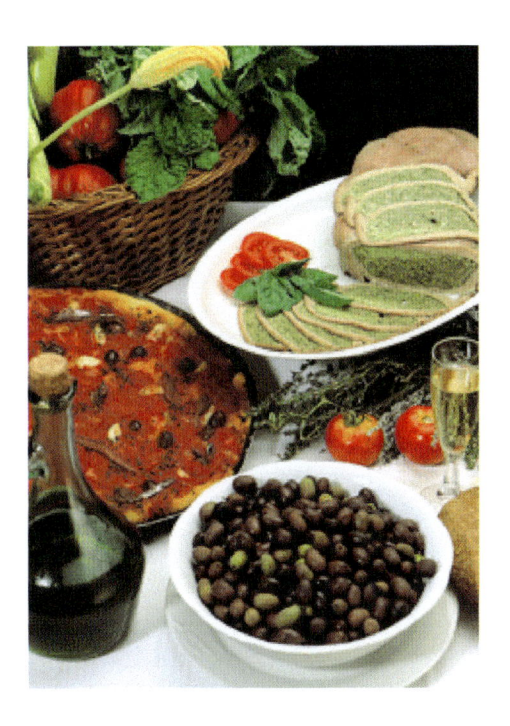

The Mediterranean Style Diet comprises pulses, fresh fruit, wholegrains, vegetables, fish, olive oil, and moderate daily wine consumption. It is low in saturated fat but high in monosaturated fatty acids. People who follow a Mediterranean Diet tend to have higher HDL cholesterol levels. The Mediterranean Diet consists of a healthy balance between omega-3 and omega-6 fatty acids. In a long term study of 423 patients who suffered a heart attack, those who followed a Mediterranean Style Diet had a 50 per cent to 70 per cent lower risk of recurrent heart disease compared with controls who received no special dietary counselling. (27)

Here is a comparison between the beneficial aspects of the cardioprotective Mediterranean Diet and the Standard American Diet.

Traditional Mediterranean Diet	Standard American Diet (SAD)
* **Cold pressed olive oil** source of vitamin E, stable when heated.	**Corn oil** highly refined damaged fat.
* **Oily fish/seafood** contains Omega-3 oils – DHA, EPA, vitamin D.	**Red Meat/dairy** high in saturated fat.
* **Pulses e.g. lentils, chick peas** providing fibre, isoflavones.	**Potatoes** high in starch, can effect blood sugar
* **Rocket, radicchio, artichoke** can aid with digestive health, appetite.	**Iceberg lettuce and cucumber** minimal nutritional value.
* **Aromatic herbs/garlic** antioxidant, antiviral and antibacterial.	**Salt** linked with blood pressure.
* **Red and yellow carotenoid rich vegetables** peppers, tomatoes. Citrus fruits rich in lycopene, limonene and vitamin C.	**Apples and bananas** imited antioxidant provision.
* **Tomato based herb sauces** lycopene rich, low fat.	**Creamy, white flour based sauces** high calorie, high fat.
* **Red wine in moderation** Source of antioxidant resveratrol.	**Spirits** no known benefits.
* **Unsalted nuts/seeds** high in zinc, vitamin E, fibre, omega-3 fats.	**Crisps** high salt content and trans-fats.

Simple cardioprotective food choices for those at risk of cardiovascular disease.

Increase consumption of:
Garlic
Porridge Oats
Oily fish – mackerel, salmon, herring
Unsalted nuts, seeds
Olive Oil
Onions
Tea, especially green tea
Blueberries, prunes, strawberries
Fruit and vegetables
Beans and pulses
Wholegrains

Reduce/Avoid consumption of:
Coffee
Fried foods
White bread, pasta
Nicotine
Biscuits, soft drinks
Excess alcohol/spirits
Excess saturated/hydrogenated fats
High sodium foods – e.g. bacon, tinned soup, pickles
Table sugar – FOS (Fructo-oligosaccharrides) powder is an ideal substitute sweetener and valuable fibre source

Exercise

Regular exercise (ideally 3 hours per week or more e.g. 30 minutes per day, 6 days per week) increases the beneficial levels of HDL cholesterol.

The importance of ridding yourself of dental amalgams

About 75 percent of adults have dangerous "silver" fillings. There is approximately 1,000 mg of mercury in the typical "silver" filling. This is nearly one million times more mercury than is present in contaminated sea food. Most people don't realize that the mercury amalgams slowly release mercury vapour. Every time you chew, mercury vapour is released and quickly finds its way into your bloodstream, where it causes oxidative processes in your tissues.

As we know oxidation is one of the main reasons you develop disease, as well as the primary reason you age. Oxidation in your body leads to inflammation, including inflammation of the lining of your blood vessels. When this occurs, your LDL levels increase as your body attempts to "patch" those damaged vessel walls with cholesterol. LDL is a carrier of cholesterol. This is why people with mercury toxicity have damaged blood vessels, and elevated cholesterol and LDL levels.

Introducing Guggul

Despite a recent trial in America by Dr Philippe O Szapary, [28] that seems to contradict the weight of evidence supporting the use of guggulipid as a cholesterol lowering herb, I want to firmly put the case for this exciting herb which I know to be very effective in lowering LDL cholesterol, raising HDL cholesterol, and lowering triglycerides.

Let's start with the history……..

An extract from the resin of the mukul myrrh tree (Commiphora mukul), guggul has been used since 600BC in Ayurvedic medicine to treat obesity and lipid disorders.

> अथर्ववेद: कां. १९ सू ३८
> न तं यक्ष्मा अरुन्धते नैनं शपथो अश्नुते।
> यं भेषजस्य गुल्गुलो: सुरभिर्गन्धो अश्नुते॥१॥
> विश्वेऽस्रस्तस्माद् यक्ष्मा मृगा अश्वा इवेरते
> यद् गुल्गुल् सैन्धवं यद् वाप्यासि समुद्रियम्॥२॥
> उभयोरग्रभं नामास्मा अरिष्टतातये॥३॥

*Original Sanskrit verse from **Atharva Veda** that refers to the medicinal values of guggul.*

Studies of guggul resulted in the publication of Satyavati's doctoral thesis entitled 'Effect of an indigenous drug on disorders of lipid metabolism with special reference to atherosclerosis and obesity (medoroga)' that was submitted to Banaras Hindu University (BHU). This pioneering work, published in 1966, provoked much interest among Indian scientists at BHU and institutions elsewhere. A number of preclinical and clinical studies were undertaken on gum guggul with emphasis on its hypolipidaemic and related properties. These were soon followed by phytochemical and pharmacognostic studies. Finally in 1988, guggulipid was available as a hypolipidaemic agent on the Indian market.

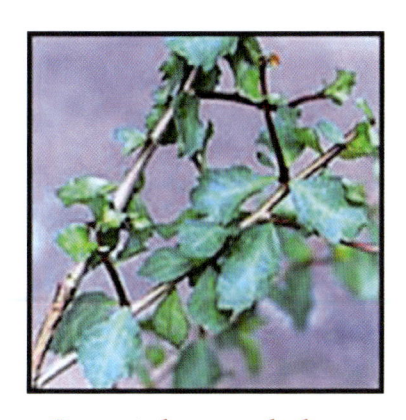

Commiphora mukul tree

What is Guggul?

Guggul is the yellowish resin (or gum) that is produced by *Commiphora mukul*, a small, thorny plant that grows throughout northern India. Guggul is also referred to as guggul gum, guggal, gugglesterone, gugulu and gum gugal. Its active components, Z-guggulsterone and E-guggulsterone, have an ability to lower both cholesterol and triglyceride levels. Specifically, guggulipid lowers VLDL and LDL cholesterol and triglycerides while simultaneously raising HDL cholesterol. This indicates guggul's primary use for providing protection against atherosclerosis. These effects are due to guggul's action on the liver which is stimulated to metabolise LDL cholesterol, effectively lowering the amount in the bloodstream.

How effective is Guggul?

Firstly on high cholesterol Studies show that 14-27% of LDL cholesterol and 22-30% of triglycerides levels were reduced when guggul was given to men and women with high cholesterol for 12 weeks with no change in diet or exercise. Several clinical studies were published in the Indian Journal of Medicine (volume 84) in 1986, Indian Pharmacopoeia and in the Journal of the Association of Physicians in India (vols 34 & 37) all stating the efficacy of guggul in lowering LDL cholesterol and triglycerides. Dr David Moore and his team at the Baylor College of Medicine in Houston found that the guggulsterone, the active ingredient in the guggul extract, blocks the activity of a receptor in the liver's cells called Farnesoid X Receptor (FXR). Later, Dr David Mangelsdorf at the University of Texas Southwestern Medical Center in Dallas confirmed that guggul blocks the receptor and affects how cholesterol is metabolised.

Secondly on atherosclerosis Guggul also appears to boost levels of 'good' cholesterol in the bloodstream, although the exact mechanism is unknown. In addition it decreases hepatic cholesterol levels and both of these actions help prevent atherosclerosis. Guggul is also an antioxidant, which helps stop the oxidization of cholesterol and the subsequent hardening of the arteries.

The following is one of many double blind randomised clinical trials conducted by scientists and healthcare professionals around the world.

Hypolipidaemic and antioxidant effects of Commiphora mukul as an adjunct to dietary therapy in patients with hypercholesterolaemia. Singh RB, Niaz MA, Ghosh S 1994 Aug, 8(4):659-64

Heart Research Laboratory, Medical Hospital and Research Centre, Moradabad, India

The effects of the administration of 50 mg of guggulipid or placebo capsules twice daily for 24 weeks were compared as adjuncts to a fruit- and vegetable-enriched prudent diet in the management of 61 patients with hypercholesterolaemia (31 in the guggulipid group and 30 in the placebo group) in a randomised, double-blind fashion. Guggulipid decreased the total cholesterol level by 11.7%, the low density lipoprotein cholesterol (LDL) by 12.5%, triglycerides by 12.0%, and the total cholesterol/high density lipoprotein (HDL) cholesterol ratio by 11.1% from the pre diet levels, whereas the levels were unchanged in the placebo group. The HDL cholesterol level showed no changes in the two groups. The lipid peroxides, indicating oxidative stress, declined 33.3% in the guggulipid group without any decrease in the placebo group. The compliance of patients was greater than 96%. The combined effect of diet and guggulipid at 36 weeks was as great as the reported lipid lowering effect of modern drugs. After a washout period of another 12 weeks, changes in blood lipoproteins were reversed in the guggulipid group without such changes in the placebo group. Side effects of guggulipid were headache, mild nausea, eructation, and hiccup in a few patients.

On a very strong personal note I know there are many clinical trials on the efficacy of guggulipid. Even in my own practice I have regularly seen patients move from a fasting triglyceride reading of 450 mg/dl to 150 mg/

dl within 12 weeks and cholesterol readings of 290 mg/dl (LDL 240/HDL 50) down to 204 mg/dl (LDL 124/HDL 80). Significantly, as compared with conventional drug therapy, no side effects were observed with my patients using guggulipid.

Important Contraindications concerning taking Guggulipid

Guggulipid has been shown to interact with CYP3A4, an enzyme system in the body that is responsible for metabolizing many chemicals, including medications. There have been reports that taking guggulipid with certain medications, such as propanolol, diltiazem, and birth control pills could reduce the effectiveness of those drugs. Conversely, taking guggulipid with other types of drugs, such as statins, may actually raise the levels of these drugs in the body, causing them to become more toxic.

Guggulipid also may increase the effectiveness of blood thinners like Coumadin (Warfarin), which may cause you to bleed more easily. This list is not limited to the drugs listed above, so if you are taking any prescription or over-the-counter medications, it would be wise not to take guggulipid, unless you are sure that an interaction between guggulipid and your medication does not exist. Additionally, you should not take guggulipid if you are pregnant or if you have a thyroid disorder, since guggulipid may lower thyroid stimulating hormone levels.

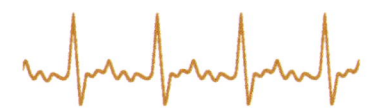

Action Plan

Be kind to your liver

Exercise regularly – aim for at least 30 minutes brisk exercise 5 days a week

Avoid hidden fats, especially saturated – check the food labels

Take supplements to lower LDL cholesterol and boost HDL cholesterol

Increase your intake of fruit, nuts, seeds and vegetables

Natural wholefoods are the best – Not processed

Garlic can ward off 'bad cholesterol' as well as vampires!

Cook the Mediterranean way

Heal your body and maintain vibrant health with optimum nutrition

Omega 3 = Oily fish – eat plenty of Salmon, Mackerel, Sardines etc

Learn ways to reduce stress

Eat a variety of foods spread out through the day

Stop smoking

Trim the fat off meat and choose lean cuts for cooking

Enjoy moderate amounts of red wine

Reduce/avoid – fried foods, saturated /hydrogenated fats and high sodium foods

Oxidised cholesterol – ensure adequate antioxidant protection

Lose any excess weight

Finally, with the right diet, relevant supplementation, exercise and stress reduction, I am certain you can make a significant impact on your health. Taking responsibility, accountability and ownership for our health is to acknowledge the precious gift of wellbeing. My heartfelt wish is that you experience vibrant health, now and long into the future.

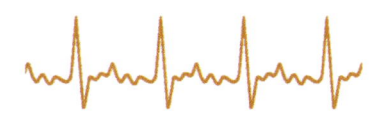

Further Reading

The Chinese Way to Health by Dr Stephen Gascoigne

Health Wars by Phillip Day

Health Defence by Dr Paul Clayton

Why Animals Don't Get Heart Attacks – But People Do by Dr Matthias Rath

The Taste That Kills and Health and Nutrition Secrets That Can Save Your Life by Russell L. Blaylock MD

What Doctors Don't Tell You by Lynne McTaggart

The Miracle Enzyme is Serrapeptase- The 2nd Gift from Silkworms by Robert Redfern

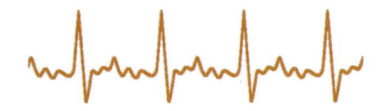

Recommended Listening

The Soul of Healing Meditations by Deepak Chopra

Power of Intention by Dr Wayne W. Dyer

About the Author

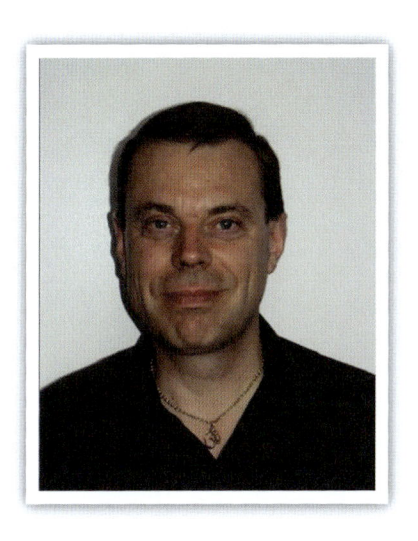

Stephen Guy-Clarke has been a passionate practitioner of natural medicine for fifteen years. He graduated in Acupuncture at the Shanghai Research Institute of Acupuncture and Meridian in 1994 and has a special interest in nutrition. Stephen has lectured and written on a number of health related topics including Asthma, 'Light, the future of Medicine' and 'You are what you absorb – The case for proper nutrition'.

Stephen also has a background in both corporate management, business ownership and technology commercialisation.

He spends his time between living in rural Suffolk, England, and beautiful Goa, India, with his wife Christine.

REFERENCES

1. Miettinen TA et al, Lancet 2: 1261, 1988

2. Sing CF et al, World Review Nut Diet 63:220-235, 1990

3. Psychol Med, 1990, 20: 785-91

4. Werbach, Dr Melvyn, Nutritional Influences on Medical Illness (Tarzana, CA: Third Line Press, 1991): 145-9.

5. Physicians' Desk Reference (Montvale, NJ: Medical Economics Data Production Company, 1995): 710-12

6. Physicians' Desk Reference: 1851-4

7. Langsjoen PH, Langsjoen AM, The clinical use of HMG CoA-reductase inhibitors and the associated depletion of coenzyme Q10. A review of animal and human publications. Biofactors 2003, 18-101-11

8. Rundek T et al, Atorvastatin decreases the coenzyme Q10 level in the blood of patients at risk for cardiovascular disease and stroke. Arch Neurol 2004, 61:889-92

9. Whitaker JM, Citizen Petition, 2002

10. Dorn, M. (1995), Improvement in Raised Lipid Levels with Artichoke Juice (Cynarascolymus), Brit J Phytotherapy, 4(1) 21-26

11. Rath Matthias, op.cit. 53

12. Kohlmeir L et al, Am J Epidemiology 146:618-628, 1997

13. Mattson FH et al, Am J Clin Nut 44:79-88, 1990

14. Ikeda et al, Lipid Research 29: 1573-1582, 1988

15. Dakenfull D, Sidhin GS, Eur J Clin Nut 44: 79-88, 1990

REFERENCES ♥ 101

16. Van Raaij JMA et al, Am J Clin Nut 35: 925-934, 1982

17. Anderson JW et al, New Eng J Med 333: 276-282, 1995

18. Sugano M et al Ann Nut Meta 28:192-199, 1984

19. Carroll KK, Fed Proc 41:2792, 1982

20. Kritchevsky D, Atherosclerosis 41:429, 1982

21. Ikeda et al, Lipid Research 29: 1573-1582, 1988

22. Oakenfull D, Sidhu GS, Eur J Clin Nut 44: 79-88, 1990

23. Mattson FH et al, Am J Clin Nut 35:697-700, 1982

24. Sirtori CR et al, Ann NY Acad Science 676: 188-201, 1993

25. Jackson RL et al, Med Res Review 13: 161-182, 1993

26. Hanninen SA et al. 'The Prevalence of Thiamine Deficiency in Hospitalized Patients With Congestive Heart Failiure', J Am Coll Cardiol 2006, 47(2): 354-61

27. Kris-Etherton P, Eckel RH, Howard BV, St. Jeor S, Bazzare TL. AHA Science Advisory: Lyon Diet Heart Study. Benefits of a Mediterranean-style, National Cholesterol Education Program/American Heart Association Step I Dietary Pattern on Cardiovascular Disease. Circulation. 2001, 103:1823.

28. Philippe O. Szapary MD, Megan L. Wolfe BS, LeAnne T. Bloedon MS, RD, Andrew J. Cucchiara PhD, Ara H. DerMarderosian PhD, Michael D. Cirigliano MD, Daniel J. Rader MD, JAMA 2003, 290:765-772.